STRENGTHENING ROAD SAFETY LEGISLATION:

A practice and resource manual for countries

DECADE OF ACTION FOR ROAD SAFETY 2011-2020

World Health Organization

WHO Library Cataloguing-in-Publication Data :

Strengthening road safety legislation: a practice and resource manual for countries.

1. *Accidents, Traffic–legislation and jurisprudence. 2.Wounds and injuries–prevention and control. 3.Safety. 4.Health promotion. 5.Handbooks. I.World Health Organization.*

ISBN 978 92 4 150510 9 *(NLM classification: WA 275)*

Graphic Design by Art'n Visual Design
Printed in Italy

CONTENTS

CHAPTER 3

CHAPTER 4

ANNEX OF LAWS

ACKNOWLEDGEMENTS

The writing and production of the manual was coordinated by Evelyn Murphy, with technical oversight and input provided by Etienne Krug, Margaret Peden and Meleckidzedeck Khayesi. We also acknowledge the input of colleagues in the World Health Organization (WHO) department of Violence and Injury Prevention and Disability: Elena Altieri, Allison Harvey, David Meddings, Thomas Shakespeare, Laura Sminkey and Tami Toroyan. Special thanks are due to Pascale Lanvers-Casasola for administrative assistance.

We acknowledge the contributions of colleagues in WHO country offices: Jonathan Passmore (Viet Nam), Victor Pavarino (Brazil), Eugenia Maria Rodriguez (WHO Regional Office for the Americas) and Francesco Zambon (the Russian Federation).

WHO gratefully acknowledges the technical contributions to this manual made by: Matts-Åke Belin, Gayle DiPietro, Moira Donahue, Anthony Greene, Gopalakrishna Gururaj, Christopher Jones, Olive Kobusingye, Luiz Otávio Maciel, Hiwote Mikonnen, Teresa Senserick, David Sleet, Kent Stevens, Sanjivi Sundar, Joël Valmain and Kiragu Wachira.

The manual also benefited from the contributions of Elizabeth Heseltine, editor, Ana Jiménez and Núria Comellas Pastallé, Art'n Visual Design graphic designers, and Ms Ann Morgan, proofreader.

Finally, WHO gratefully acknowledges the financial contributions from Bloomberg Philanthropies that made preparation and publication of this manual possible.

INTRODUCTION

On World Health Day 2004, which was dedicated to road traffic safety, the World Health Organization (WHO) and the World Bank launched the *World report on road traffic injury prevention (1)*, which describes the global burden of road traffic injuries. The aim of the report was to encourage governments and other stakeholders to address the issue of road traffic crashes and their consequences. The *World report* also set out a comprehensive approach to reducing injury and death resulting from crashes and urged governments to take specific action to prevent road traffic crashes, minimize injuries and their consequences and evaluate the effect of these activities, which should include setting and enforcing:

- speed limits appropriate to the function of the road;
- laws requiring seat-belts or child restraints for all motor vehicle occupants;
- laws requiring riders of bicycles and motorized two-wheelers to wear helmets;
- blood alcohol limits for drivers, with random breath-testing at check-points *(1)*.

The first WHO *Global status report on road safety (2)*, published in 2009 and summarizing data supplied by 178 countries, documents recent efforts made by countries to improve their road safety record. It also provides benchmarks against which countries can compare their road safety measures and recommends a range of activities, both regulatory and non-regulatory, that could be undertaken. Comprehensive legislation—which incorporates strict, appropriate penalties, backed by consistent, sustained enforcement and public education—has been proven to be a strong catalyst for changing behaviour, norms and public perceptions about road safety *(2, 3)*. The 2009 report revealed that legislation on the known risk factors for road traffic injuries is incomplete in the majority of countries (85%) and that the existing laws are often inadequately enforced, particularly in low- and middle-income countries. The second *Global status report on road safety (4)*, published in March 2013 shows no overall improvement in the number of countries that have comprehensive road safety legislation.

In May 2010, the United Nations General Assembly approved resolution 64/255 *(5)*, proclaiming a 'Decade of Action for Road Safety 201–2020', which calls on Member States to take 'joint multisectoral action to increase the proportion of countries with comprehensive legislation on key risk factors for road traffic injuries... to 50 percent by the end of the Decade...'. In April 2012, the General Assembly approved resolution 66/260 *(6)*, which 'Encourages Member States that have not yet done so, to adopt and implement national road safety legislation and regulations on the major risk factors, and improve implementation through social marketing campaigns and consistent and sustained enforcement activities.'

This manual, *Strengthening road safety legislation*, describes methods and resources that practitioners and decision-makers can use for enacting new laws or regulations or amending existing ones as part of a comprehensive road safety strategy. In particular, it recommends adopting a stepwise approach to assessing and improving legislation relating to five specific risk factors for road traffic injuries, as well as to post-crash care. It can therefore be used to:

- develop an understanding of the framework of legislation and relevant processes that are applicable in a country;
- review current national legislation and regulations and identify barriers to the implementation and enforcement of effective road safety measures;

- identify available resources, such as international agreements, and evidence-based guidance and recommendations on effective measures, to improve legislation;
- prepare action plans to strengthen national legislation and regulations for the five main risk factors and for post-crash care, including advocating for improvement.

There are a number of other important topics, aside from those relating to the key risk factors for road traffic injuries and post-crash care discussed here, that need to be addressed to achieve a comprehensive national system of road safety legislation and regulation; however, they are beyond the scope of this manual. They include, vehicle and helmet manufacturing standards and testing, third-party insurance, victim's rights and compensation, graduated driver licensing systems, road audits and design standards and driving hours for commercial drivers.

References

1. Peden M et al., eds. *World report on road traffic injury prevention.* Geneva, World Health Organization, 2004.
2. *Global status report on road safety: time for action.* Geneva, World Health Organization, 2009.
3. Zaal D. *Traffic law enforcement: a review of the literature.* Melbourne, Monash University Accident Research Centre, 1994 (Report No. 53).
4. *Global status report on road safety 2013: supporting a decade of action.* Geneva, World Health Organization, 2013.
5. Resolution A/RES/64/255. Improving Global Road Safety. Sixty-fourth session of the United Nations General Assembly, New York, 10 May 2010 (http://www.un.org/en/ga/64/resolutions.shtml, accessed 6 June 2013).
6. Resolution A/RES/66/260. Improving Global Road Safety. Sixty-sixth session of the United Nations General Assembly, New York, 23 May 2012 (http://www.un.org/en/ga/66/resolutions.shtml, accessed 6 June 2013).

Chapter 1

A legal framework for road safety laws and regulations

Chapter 1 A legal framework for road safety laws and regulations

Comprehensive national road safety laws and regulations are effective in reducing injuries and fatalities among all road users. Enacting such laws is, however, influenced by various factors, not least of which are political will, resource capacity and challenges in changing road user behaviour. It is important to understand not only the forms of road safety laws and regulations but also the context within which legislative changes can be made.

1.1 Laws and regulations relevant to road safety

The terminology used in this manual to distinguish between regulatory instruments was adapted from various sources. Hence:

- A **law** or **legislation** is a mandate or standard enacted by a national law-making body or parliament at state or federal level. It is enforceable, with positive or negative consequences of noncompliance. In some countries, the term used is an **act** or **decree**.

- A **bill** is a draft piece of legislation introduced and published in accordance with the procedures of the country for consideration by a parliament or equivalent legislative organ of government, at state or federal level; as it is not yet approved, a bill is not yet law.

- A **regulation** or **rule** is a statement of policy or guideline promulgated by executive branches of government, such as ministries, to further define or clarify a law. It has the force and effect of a law.

- An **ordinance** or **by-law** is a law set by municipal or other local government. Although it is not national, it is sometimes heavily influenced by national law. Local ordinances can result in a harmonized system when they mirror national laws, or they can result in fragmentation when localities and municipalities are given broad powers and do not align with national laws. While the focus of this manual is on federal and national laws, some local examples are given.

- A **standard** is technical documentation that sets forth minimum safety requirements that apply nationally, such as standards for motorcycle helmets and child restraints. A standard can also define how a law or regulation is to be implemented at local level; e.g. local authorities can set speed limits in built-up areas, construction areas or near schools, usually within national limits.

The type of road safety law depends on whether a country has a federal or a national system. States may have different degrees of flexibility to enact laws that are different from federal or national laws. For example, in Australia, India and the United States of America, where there are federal systems, states can enact their own laws, which can give rise to differing road safety standards within the same country. Furthermore, in some countries, local governments and municipalities can also enact their own laws.

The laws relevant to road safety vary from country to country, sometimes depending on the type of behaviour or action they are intended to address. For example:

- **Transport** or **motor vehicle** laws address topics such as driving privileges, licensing and vehicle registration, road signs and signalling, driving conduct, motor vehicle manufacturing standards and commercial driver working hours. Such laws are not limited to safety on the roads but can include transport infrastructure.

- **Criminal** laws criminalize certain behaviours, such as careless driving, reckless driving and driving under the influence of alcohol or drugs.

- **Insurance** laws address drivers' liability and the compensation of road crash victims, such as payments for property damage or medical costs.

- **Constitutional** laws in some jurisdictions address the rights of people to health care, including emergency treatment.

- **Public health** laws can include topics such as post-crash interventions, ranging from access to and provision of care in hospitals to protection of first responders.

- **Tort** laws, within civil law, determine liability by assigning fault based on driving behaviour. Tort laws and litigation history can define or guide how fault is assigned and who will be responsible for compensating the victims. These laws can deter people from engaging in actions or behaviour that can harm others and can encourage responsible action *(1)*. General prerequisites for liability under tort laws include.

- *Breach of a 'legal duty'*: The action or inaction that resulted in harm must be something that a reasonable person would not be expected to do, such as going through a red light.
- *Causation:* A causal association between the action (or omission) and the harm must be demonstrated, such as failure to stop at a red light (omission) and striking a pedestrian.
- *Harm:* The result of the act (or omission) must result in harm in order for litigation or liability to be initiated. This element is often referred to as 'damages' to the victim, such as compensating for loss of earnings resulting from permanent or temporary absence from work or loss of support by a dependent *(2)*.

Box 1.1 summarizes the legal framework and types of laws relevant to road safety in India.

1.2 Factors that influence legislative action on road safety

Despite the existence of national road safety laws and historical precedence, it is difficult to pinpoint what motivates or initiates legislative action at a national level. While traffic statistics can often spur legislation, they are not the only driving forces; other factors include, political will and high-level commitment (especially for legal reform), public pressure, a personal road-related tragedy in a law-maker's family, and changes in social norms and values. Global

Box 1.1 Legal framework and types of laws relevant to road safety in India

INDIA'S MOTOR VEHICLE ACT 1988 is the national law governing road safety, covering issues such as driver licensing and user behaviour *(3)*. The Central Motor Vehicles Rules of 1989 are the implementing regulations to the law *(4)*. The Act gives state governments the authority to adopt their own rules to put into practice certain provisions, thereby resulting in differences in implementation from state to state. A bill was proposed recently to amend the Motor Vehicle Act to increase fines *(5)*.

The Indian Penal Code criminalizes reckless and dangerous driving under the road safety laws. Thus, driving in a 'rash and negligent' manner that endangers the life or personal safety of others or causes injury can be prosecuted as homicide, murder or negligence resulting in death. In addition, under road safety laws in India, individuals who drive at a speed or in a manner that puts the public in danger or those driving with a blood alcohol concentration above the limit can be imprisoned for anywhere between 6 months (for a first offence) and 3 years (for a second offence), or pay a fine or be subject to both a fine and imprisonment *(6, 7)*.

The Motor Vehicle Act also requires that drivers carry liability insurance to cover injuries or damage to any property or death arising out of the use of a vehicle *(7)*. Third-party insurance is regulated by the Insurance Regulatory and Development Authority, which also reviews claims and premium rates *(8)*.

Road traffic crashes have been the subject of tort cases. Before enactment of the Motor Vehicle Act in 1988—which was a revision of a 1939 law—liability in road traffic crashes was resolved as a matter of fault in court under tort law. The 1988 Act, subsequent amendments in 1994 and court cases have since defined liability more strictly *(9)*. Before 1988, liability in vehicle crashes was based predominantly on fault. With the 1988 Act, the owner was held strictly liable when the crash resulted in permanent dismemberment or death, and the amount of compensation was regulated. The 1994 amendment imposes stricter liability on the person who caused the injury, and the insurance company is obliged to pay a certain amount to the victim or the victim's heirs, regardless of who is at fault.

commitment and recommendations on best practice from international policy-making and technical institutions such as the United Nations can also prompt the reform of road safety laws. Legislation is an important part of a comprehensive road safety strategy to help countries to reduce injuries and fatalities and achieve overall goals for road safety.

International regulations serve as benchmarks and can provide a legal framework on which regions and countries can base evidence-based practice. For example, the United Nations *Conventions on Road Traffic of 1949 and 1968 (10)* and the *Convention on Road Signs and Signals of 1968 (11)* recommend best practices for countries, particularly in the European region. The *Consolidated Resolution on Road Traffic (12)*, which supplements the *Convention on Road Traffic 1968*, and the *European Agreement of 1971 (13)* provide guidance on improving road safety and a framework for greater voluntary harmonization of regulations at international level.

1.2.1 Recent trends in injuries and fatalities

A heavy toll on human lives, such as increasing trends in fatalities and injuries tends to draw attention to road safety. Global attention has been focused on the need to reduce injuries and fatalities by publication of the estimated annual numbers of road injuries and deaths and in particular by WHO's forecasted increase in the ranking of road injuries as a leading cause of death, from ninth place in 2004 to fifth place in 2020 if no action is taken *(14)*.

Countries must maintain an efficient, comprehensive system for managing information on road traffic injuries and fatalities, as these statistics significantly influence policy and legislation. Policy-makers require data disaggregated by, for example, type of road user, risk behaviour and geographical region, so that they are relevant to the locale and to the legislative issues being considered.

1.2.2 Social norms and values

A social norm is 'a concept from social psychology that refers to implicit rules or standards inferred by individuals from the behaviour they observe or expectations they assume in their social milieu and that guide their own behaviour; they can be descriptive—in other words how most people behave—or injunctive—how others think one should behave' *(15)*. Laws and regulations can change the social meaning attributed to certain behaviour and can change individual behaviour. Social meaning can be changed by law, by categorizing and regulating behaviour by what is acceptable and what is not. Behaviour can be changed by requiring certain actions, such as wearing a seat-belt, or by requiring people to refrain from certain actions, such as drinking and driving.

In order that such laws or regulations are passed, law-makers and regulatory bodies must be motivated to act. Equally important is public support for laws and regulations, especially when the legislation imposed curtails—to a certain extent—personal liberty, beliefs and social norms. Thus, the extent to which law-makers in a country are willing and able to regulate personal activities such as driving may depend on personal values and how citizens, the law-makers themselves and the government balance personal liberties against public good *(16, 17)*. The perceptions of the public and individuals of their duties and responsibilities with regard to the community as a whole and the extent to which they are willing to give up certain elements of personal freedom to protect society can influence road safety laws *(18)*.

1.2.3 Financial, human and other resources

Both financial and human resources play significant roles in legislation. Although legislation is often the basis for budget allocations, the allocations may not match the mandates, making implementation virtually impossible.

In some countries, an economic impact assessment is required before new legislation is enacted. For example, in Australia, a 'regulation impact statement' is required for any regulatory proposal that is likely to affect the business or the not-for-profit sector, unless the impact would be minor and would not substantially change existing arrangements. The regulation impact statement is based on an in-depth analysis, consideration of alternative proposals and an analysis of costs and benefits.

The elements that must be addressed include:

- the problem or issues that gave rise to the proposed legislation;
- the objective(s);
- the viable regulatory and non-regulatory options for achieving the objective(s);
- an assessment of the impact of each option (costs, benefits and, when relevant, levels of risk) on consumers, business, government and the community;
- a consultation statement;
- a recommended option;
- a strategy to implement and review the recommended option *(19)*.

Taking motorcycle helmets as an example, any new law or regulation should take into account the cost of designing and testing helmets and the consequent price range of helmets, which will affect compliance and ultimately the effectiveness of this intervention. If people cannot afford to buy helmets and there is no programme for distributing them, they will not comply with the regulation. In Egypt, it has not been possible to introduce policies and legislation for mandatory child restraints for cost reasons *(20)*. Other interventions require government investment, such as police training, enforcement activities and improving infrastructure. Often, a government decides not to legislate an intervention only on the basis of its cost, without taking into account the avoidable costs to families after a crash.

It is important to weigh the cost of implementing an intervention against the cost of not implementing it. This can include a comparison of the medical costs related to injuries and the economic costs of lost productivity with the costs of implementation, such as increasing police capacity to enforce the law or the purchase and installation of instruments like speed cameras. Box 1.2 gives estimates of the number of lives saved and the economic costs associated with introducing a seat-belt law in Canada.

Box 1.2 Lives saved and economic benefits of seat-belt use in Canada

SEAT-BELTS are one of the most effective road safety interventions: wearing a seat-belt reduces the risk of ejection from a vehicle and suffering serious or fatal injury by 40–65%, and their use is extremely cost-effective to society. In Canada, the lives of about 8600 drivers and front-seat passengers were saved by seat-belts between 1990 and 1997. The economic savings attributed to the use of seat-belts during this period were estimated to be about 12.9 billion Canadian dollars, taking into consideration factors such as the lost productivity of people who might otherwise have been injured in a road traffic crash. When the analysis was extended to 2000, it was estimated that 11 690 motor vehicle occupant lives were saved, with an estimated 17.5 billion Canadian dollars in economic benefits *(21)*.

1.3 Influence of different sectors on road safety laws and regulations

Whatever the rationale for initiating legislation, multiple sectors should be involved in its development. Legislation is not just the work of parliamentarians or lawmakers: getting laws passed also requires collaboration among government agencies, nongovernmental organizations, civil society, the media, advocacy groups and private organizations. Some examples of the involvement of different sectors in bringing about legislative change at the national level are listed below:

- In Mexico, reforms to the drink–driving law in Guadalajara in 2010 and a change in people's perspectives about drink–driving came about largely because of a change in the name of the law, from *Ley Antiborrachos* (Anti-drunk Law) to *Ley Salvavidas* (Lifeguard Law), the participation of civil society, technical guidance from the WHO Regional Office for the Americas (which provided evidence in support of the law reform) and constant media involvement.

- The *'Por Amor'* seat-belt campaign in Costa Rica during 2003–2004 was organized collaboratively by the Ministry of Transport, the National Road Safety Council, the National Insurance Institute and the Automobile Club, with support from the FIA Foundation for the Automobile and Society Foundation. The campaign, with stricter law enforcement, brought about lasting changes in the seat-belt law *(22)*.

- In the United Kingdom a parliamentary committee, the Parliamentary Advisory Council for Transport Safety, was responsible for introducing legislation for front seat-belt use in the 1980s, followed some years later by the introduction of speed humps and rear seat-belts *(23)*.

- Victims' organizations can draw attention to the human toll of road traffic crashes to bring about legislative changes. The UK-based Brake charity issued a report in 2011 on the impact of road traffic crashes on families and the lack of appropriate government support, showing that about 500 families are affected each year by such events. Brake called *for* a law recognizing the needs of families bereaved due to road traffic crashes and for integrated support for victims by the criminal justice system and others *(24)*.

1.4 Importance of timing in bringing about change

Despite the evidence of research and forecasted increases in road traffic injuries and fatalities, appropriate legal measures are not always adopted immediately, partly because many other factors influence national road safety legislation. The road safety community must therefore be ready to push for change at a national level when the opportunity presents itself.

The 'multiple streams' framework creates a scenario in which action is taken at the point in time at which three steams converge:

- *problem stream:* the extent to which an issue is viewed as a problem;

- *policy stream:* the effectiveness of countermeasures;

- *politics stream:* community demand for action and acceptance of countermeasures *(25)*.

Understanding these streams might lead to a strategy for bringing about change when the time is ripe, as illustrated by the change in Australia's novice driver policy (Box 1.3).

1.5 Resources for bringing about change

Many guidelines and recommendations provide information that is helpful for designing national road safety laws and regulations. A number of international legal instruments, agreements and normative guides give models of comprehensive legislation and regulation to improve road safety and to promote action. Regional and global reports also reflect evolving practices and evidence on the most effective ways of reducing injuries and fatalities. Countries can use such information to assess their own existing road safety legislation and to determine how it can be strengthened, by comparing their own laws with others. The documents can also provide the political and societal impetus for action on road safety legislation.

The United Nations Economic Commission for Europe (UNECE) Working Party on Road Traffic published their *Consolidated Resolution on Road Traffic* in 2010 *(12)*, which describes measures and practices that states can implement voluntarily as well as specific recommendations on safe speed thresholds by road type, drink–driving (including for novice drivers), driving under the influence of other (non-alcoholic) substances that affect driving capacity, use of seat-belts and child restraint systems, use of mobile phones and other risk factors.

WHO's *World report on road traffic injury prevention (26)* recommends that governments enact and enforce legislation to require the use of seat-belts and child restraints and the wearing of motorcycle and bicycle helmets, and to prevent alcohol-impaired driving.

Another WHO publication, *Youth and road safety (28)*, provides information about road traffic injuries in young people. It also includes evidence-based strategies to reduce some of the risk factors for road traffic-related injuries and fatalities among young people, such as lowering the blood alcohol limit for novice drivers and the use of child restraints.

Box 1.3 Factors that influenced policies on novice drivers in Australia

A VARIETY OF FACTORS that affected policies on novice drivers in four states in Australia between 2007 and 2009 were identified from interviews with people involved in the debate. The factors that favoured the policies included:

- a increasing body of evidence from other jurisdictions showing the effectiveness of the policies;
- dissemination of evidence by researchers, lobbying and advocacy by influential stakeholders and media reporting of multiple fatalities in crashes involving novice drivers;
- international and domestic research on restrictions on night driving and peer passengers, which raised support for the policies among influential nongovernment groups, such as motoring groups and professional road safety advocates.

Factors that slowed policy changes included:

- opposition by politicians and other senior public servants, who perceived the policies as unpopular in the community and unfeasible politically;
- concern that the restrictions would undermine designated driver programmes, in which one driver remains sober to transport others consuming alcohol;
- issues of mobility and social equity.

The conclusion of the study was that the Australian graduated driver licensing policy can be acted on only if adequate political support is available, in response to community demand for action and public acceptance of similar policies in neighbouring states *(27)*. Researchers might therefore raise community support for unpopular but evidence-based policies during policy reform.

The *2013 Global status report on road safety (29)* recommends that governments pass comprehensive laws to protect all road users, by setting speed limits appropriate to the type and function of each road, stipulating blood alcohol limits that help reduce drink-driving, and requiring the use of appropriate protective measures. It further recommends that existing legislation be reviewed and amended to conform to good practice based on sound evidence of effectiveness. It provides evidence for the effectiveness of speed thresholds, blood alcohol limits, wearing of seat-belts and use of appropriate child restraints and helmets.

WHO and some members of the United Nations Road Safety Collaboration (the World Bank, the FIA Foundation for the Automobile and Society, and the Global Road Safety Partnership), an informal consultative mechanism whose members are committed to road safety efforts and in particular to the implementation of the recommendations of the *World report on road traffic injury prevention (26)*, have published a series of manuals for decision-makers and practitioners that provide practical advice for reducing the incidence of road traffic crashes:

- *Helmets: a road safety manual for decision-makers and practitioners (30);*
- *Drinking and driving: a road safety manual for decision-makers and practitioners (31);*
- *Speed management: a road safety manual for decision-makers and practitioners (32);*
- *Seat-belts and child restraints: a road safety manual for decision-makers and practitioners (33).*

These manuals describe the steps relevant to each country to bring out policy change and provide practical advice on implementation of effective measures to address these risk factors. They include technical measures and the institutional structures required for interventions against risks associated with speeding, drinking and driving, not wearing seat-belts or helmets, and not transporting children in child restraints.

Resources and guidance for other areas of road safety policy and legislation include distractions while driving and driving under the influence of drugs. *Mobile phone use: a growing problem of driver distraction (34)* presents evidence that use of a mobile phone while driving distracts drivers and also describes legislative measures being taken to address this growing problem. While it reveals some inconsistencies in the legislation and provides no specific recommendations or guidelines, it sets out some of the arguments, practices and legislation being put into place in countries that are ready to tackle this issue.

While it is known that substances other than alcohol reduce driving capacity, there is no authoritative, complete list of such substances. As a result, there is no evidence-based recommendation on driving under the influence of substances other than alcohol. The International Council on Alcohol, Drugs and Traffic Safety lists psychoactive drugs according to whether their use can safely be combined with driving a car *(35)*. These categories are:

- *Drugs presumed to be safe or unlikely to produce an effect:* the advice is 'Be careful not to drive before having read the warnings in the package insert.'
- *Drugs likely to have minor or moderate adverse effects:* the advice is 'Do not drive without consulting a health care professional about the possible impairing effects.'
- *Drugs likely to have severe effects or presumed to be potentially dangerous:* the advice is 'Do not drive when taking this drug, and consult a health care professional about starting to drive again after evaluation of the treatment outcomes.'

The recommendation of the UNECE Working Party on Road Safety *(12)* is that governments should encourage research and exchange of best practices to arrive at a common classification of substances that affect driving capacity, and enact legislation to prevent driving under the influence of such substances.

Large reductions in the number of deaths and cases of serious injury can be achieved by adopting a holistic 'Safe system' approach to road traffic safety *(36)*. This approach is based on evidence-based activities supported by appropriate organizational management capacity. It is an aspirational model, with the long-term objective of eliminating deaths and serious injuries due to traffic crashes. Areas of legislation that must be addressed to move 'towards zero' include: regulation of road-user behaviour, with clear, mandatory rules and sanctions for noncompliance; regulation of infrastructure, covering road systems design and construction that conform to best safety practice; and vehicle standards *(37)*.

Chapter 3 provides regulatory measures for addressing each of the five known risk factors for road traffic injuries and advice on establishing appropriate regulation to address post-crash care.

1.6 References

1. Brown C. Deterrence in tort and no-fault: the New Zealand experience. *California Law Review*, 1995, 73:976–1002.

2. Satchwell K. Tort claims for road accident compensation and social security in South Africa. *International Social Security Association Review*, 2004, 57:111–132.

3. *Motor Vehicles Act 1988*. New Delhi, Ministry of Road Transport and Highways, 1988 (http://www.morth.nic.in/index2.asp?slid=95&sublinkid=54&lang=1, accessed 9 January 2013).

4. *Central Motor Vehicles Rules 1989*. New Delhi, Ministry of Road Transport and Highways, 1989 (http://www.morth.nic.in/index2.asp?slid=99&sublinkid=58&lang=1, accessed 9 January 2013).

5. Dipak KD. Cabinet OKs tougher penalties under Motor Vehicle Act. *The Times of India*, 1 March 2012 (http://articles.timesofindia.indiatimes.com/2012-03-01/india/31112816_1_fines-first-offence-jail-term, accessed 9 January 2013).

6. *Indian Penal Code 1860*, Sections 279, 336, 337 and 338. New Delhi, Ministry of Law and Justice (http://indiacode.nic.in/, accessed 9 January 2013).

7. *Indian Motor Vehicles Act 1988*, Sections 146, 147, 184 and 185. New Delhi, Ministry of Law and Justice (http://indiacode.nic.in/, accessed 9 January 2013).

8. *Annual report 2011–2012*, New Delhi, Insurance Regulatory Development Authority, 2012 (http://www.irda.gov.in/ADMINCMS/cms/frmGeneral_NoYearList.aspx?DF=AR&mid=11.1, accessed 9 January 2013).

9. Singh R. *Relationship between liability regimes and economic development: A study of motor vehicle accidents in India*. New Delhi, Centre for the Study of Law and Governance, Jawaharlal Nehru University, 2009 (CSLG /WP/09/03).

10. *Convention on Road Traffic, of 19 September 1949 and 8 November 1968*. Geneva, United Nations Economic Commission for Europe.

11. *Convention on Road Signs and Signals, of 8 November 1968. Geneva, United Nations Economic Commission for Europe.*

12. *Consolidated Resolution on Road Traffic, 14 August 2009* (ECE/TRANS/WP.1/123). Geneva, United Nations Economic Commission for Europe, Working Party on Road Traffic Safety, 2010.

13. *European agreement supplementing the 1968 Convention on Road Traffic, of 1 May 1971. Geneva, United Nations Economic Commission for Europe.*

14. *Global status report on road safety: time for action*. Geneva, World Health Organization, 2009.

15. Gielen AC, Sleet DA, Green LW. Community models and approaches for intervention. In: Gielen AC, Sleet DA, DiClemente RJ, eds. *Injury and violence prevention*. Jossey-Bass, 2006:65–82.

16. Ross HL. The Scandinavian myth: the effectiveness of drinking-and-driving in Sweden and Norway. *Journal of Legal Studies*, 1975, 4:285–310.

17. Jessop G. Victoria's unique approach to road safety: a history of government regulation. *Australian Journal of Politics and History*, 2009, 55:190–200.

18. Zambon F. The subtle trade-off between personal freedom and social responsibility. *Journal of Epidemiology and Community Health*, 2008, 62:90.

19. Department of Finance and Deregulation. *Australian Government regulatory impact statement*. Canberra, Office of Best Practice Regulation, 2010 (http://www.finance.gov.au/obpr/ris/gov-ris.html, accessed 9 January 2013).

20. *The EU-Twinning expertise for enhancing road safety in Egypt: Germany, Austria, Egypt 2008–2011* (Twinning Project No. EG08/AA/TP13) (http://www.svpt.uni-wuppertal.de/fileadmin/bauing/svpt/Publikationen/The_Twinning_Expertise_for_Enhancing_Road_Safety_in_Egypt_01.pdf, accessed 9 January 2013).

21. Road Safety Directorate and Motor Vehicle Regulation Directorate. *Evaluation of the effectiveness of air bags and seat-belts: estimates of lives saved among front seat occupants of light-duty vehicles involved in collisions attributable to the use of seat-belts and air bags in Canada. A follow up.* Ottawa, Transport Canada, Minister of Public Works and Government Services, 2001 (TP No. 13187E, Fact sheet RS 2001–03 E).

22. *Por amor: Costa Rica's seat-belt campaign.* London, FIA Foundation for the Automobile and Society, 2005 (http://www.fiafoundation.org/news/archive/2006/Pages/CostaRicanseatbeltcampaignwinsinternationalroadsafetyaward.aspx, accessed 9 January 2013).

23. Allsop R. *Road safety: Britain in Europe.* London, Parliamentary Advisory Council for Transport Safety, 2001.

24. Casey L. *Review into the needs of families bereaved by homicide.* London, Ministry of Justice, 2011 (http://www.brake.org.uk/latest-news/060711.htm, accessed 9 January 2013).

25. Kingdon JW. *Agendas, alternatives, and public policies. Update edition, with an epilogue on health care, 2/E.* Washington, DC, Pearson Education, 2011.

26. Peden M et al., eds. *World report on road traffic injury prevention.* Geneva, World Health Organization, 2004.

27. Hichcliff R, Poulos R, Invers RQ, Senserrick T. Understanding novice driver policy agenda setting. *Public Health*, 2011, 125*(4)*:217–221.

28. Peden M, Toroyan T, eds. *Youth and road safety.* Geneva, World Health Organization, 2007.

29. *Global status report on road safety: supporting a decade of action.* Geneva, World Health Organization, 2013.

30. *Helmets: a road safety manual for decision-makers and practitioners.* Geneva, World Health Organization, 2006.

31. *Drinking and driving: a road safety manual for decision-makers and practitioners.* Geneva, Global Road Safety Partnership, 2007.

32. *Speed management: a road safety manual for decision-makers and practitioners.* Geneva, Global Road Safety Partnership, 2008.

33. *Seat-belts and child restraints: a road safety manual for decision-makers and practitioners.* London, FIA Foundation for the Automobile and Society, 2009.

34. *Mobile phone use: a growing problem of driver distraction.* Geneva, World Health Organization, 2011.

35. Verster JC, Mets MAJ. Psychoactive medication and traffic safety. *International Journal of Environmental Research and Public Health*, 2009, 6:1041–1054.

36. *Road traffic safety management systems.* Geneva, International Organization for Standardization, 2012, (http://www.iso.org/iso/iso_catalogue/catalogue_tc/catalogue_tc_browse.htm?commid=558313, accessed 9 January 2013).

37. International Transport Forum. *Towards zero: ambitious road safety targets and the safe systems approach.* Paris, Organisation for Economic Co-operation and Development, 2008.

Chapter 2

Assessing and improving laws and regulations

Chapter 2 Assessing and improving laws and regulations

An assessment of laws and regulations ensures:

- a clear picture of current laws and regulations in order to identify any gaps;
- that laws and regulations are not changed without a clear understanding of the country's needs;
- the support of stakeholders for any necessary changes to laws and regulations.

Countries can assess and improve laws and regulations by following steps in Table 2.1 to address five major risk factors (speed, seat-belt use, drink–driving and use of helmets and child restraints) and post-crash care.

Table 2.1 Assessment of laws and regulations

Step 1	**Conduct an institutional assessment**
	Identify the national and state or provincial bodies responsible for road safety and their roles and responsibilities with respect to initiating and implementing legislation and regulation.
Step 2	**Review national laws and regulations**
	Review all existing national road safety laws and regulations and any amendments being prepared.
Step 3	**Assess gaps in laws and regulations**
	▪ Are there inconsistent or conflicting provisions in the law?
	▪ Are there too many exclusions and exceptions to the law or regulation?
	▪ Do laws or regulations cover all the risk factors?
	▪ What challenges do the problems identified present to enforcement?
	▪ Can the provisions of the law be implemented or enforced?
	▪ Does the law achieve the purpose for which it was enacted, on the basis of data analysis and other information?
Step 4	**Assess the comprehensiveness of laws and regulations**
	Assess comprehensiveness for the five main risk factors:
	▪ Are they based on evidence?
	▪ Do they include enforcement provisions?
	▪ Do they include appropriate penalties?
	Assess the comprehensiveness of laws and regulations relating to post-crash care, bearing in mind it is part of a wider system of trauma care in a country:
	▪ Conduct a rapid assessment of the institutional framework for trauma care.
	▪ Ensure that laws and regulations address the topics generally covered in a mature trauma care system.

2.1 Conducting an institutional assessment

Part of an institutional assessment involves identifying the government ministries or institutions that are directly responsible for road safety (or the activities of which affect road safety), and determining their roles and responsibilities with respect to laws and regulations.

In general, national laws establish the framework for road safety and confer the responsibility for drafting detailed regulations to a ministry or regulatory body with the appropriate technical expertise, and the responsibility for enforcement to another government body, such as the police, and ultimately the judiciary, such as traffic courts and criminal courts. Various sectors of local government may set local laws and decide how national laws are implemented locally. Sectors that usually play a role in road safety management include:

- transport and licensing (roads and motor vehicles);
- health;
- police;
- justice;
- education (training and licensing);
- private sector business and commerce;
- industry standard-setting entities (e.g. standards for vehicles, motorcycle helmets, child restraints).

National agencies that are empowered to regulate various aspects of road safety or to allocate resources should be involved (Box 2.1). Including licensing bodies, such as for alcohol, could help to change national laws nationally and locally.

In addition to reviewing the roles and responsibilities of ministries and other government bodies, the assessment may also address how effective and coordinated these bodies are in meeting their responsibilities, their resources and capacity to discharge their duties, and whether their composition or structure is suitable for their operation. The legal and administrative framework of the institutions might also have to be reviewed to determine whether it allows them to meet their responsibilities. Thus, a comprehensive institutional assessment comprises not only identification of national bodies involved in road safety legislation and regulation, but also developing an understanding of what they do and how well they are doing it, as well as their strengths, weaknesses and needs.

Box 2.1 Intersectoral collaboration: Viet Nam's national traffic safety committee

VIET NAM'S NATIONAL TRAFFIC SAFETY COMMITTEE, formed in 1997, is a legislative advisory body to the Prime Minister on transport safety issues. This committee, with membership from several ministries, was instrumental in preparing and implementing motorcycle helmet legislation in 2007. The committee coordinated introduction of the legislation, with the individual ministries having the following roles:

The Ministry of Transport coordinated preparation of the legislation and instructed other members of the committee and the 63 provincial traffic safety committees on implementing the law.

The Ministry of Public Security gave instruction to all police in the country to ensure that the law was enforced.

The Ministry of Health set up a hospital surveillance system for road traffic injuries, including head injuries.

The Ministry of Education and Training provided school courses on the benefits of wearing a helmet.

The Ministry of Communication and Information delivered social marketing through official channels and the mass media, including daily road safety programmes on national television.

Source: reference *(1)*.

2.2 Reviewing national laws and regulations

The compilation and review of all national road safety laws and regulations (plus any amendments under consideration) is the first step towards identifying gaps and areas of law or regulation that should be strengthened. The questions that can be asked in conducting such a high-level review are:

- What is the formal title and complete citation of the law or regulation? Some laws are commonly referred to by names such as 'The Traffic Act', while others are known by the name of the member of parliament who sponsored it.
- Is the law or regulation national or subnational (e.g. state or provincial)?
- What is the date of enactment (or amendment) and the effective date? This can be useful if a recent law or regulation has not yet taken effect or for assessing whether a law or regulation was phased in, for example, by stepwise enforcement of provisions.
- What road safety issues are addressed in the law or regulation?
- Are there laws or regulations governing pre-hospital trauma care (e.g. emergency medical system or emergency access number), certification or licensure, education and training of post-crash care providers, licensing standards for hospital-based care (e.g. tertiary care facility requirements) or quality assurance (e.g. mandatory reporting requirements)?
- Does the text of the law authorize a specialized agency (e.g. ministry of transport, health or interior, a national board, a body responsible for standards development) to draft regulations? If it does, determine whether a regulation was drafted and when it became effective. Also determine whether national or subnational entities have the authority to set different standards (e.g. a law mandates a speed limit of 80–100 km/h, but local governments can set speed limits within this range.)
- Who is responsible for enforcement?
- Has legislative or regulatory change been recommended in any national (or subnational) plans or reports?

Sometimes, a government or parliament establishes a body to review laws. For example, in India, the government set up the Sundar Expert Committee to conduct a comprehensive review of the India Motor Vehicles Act, 1988. The report submitted to the Ministry of Road Transport and Highways in 2011 made a number of recommendations, with a rationale for the proposed changes *(2)*. The work of similar government bodies can be a good source of information on road safety laws and regulation.

If the review is the first of its kind to be conducted, there will be a large volume of documents on a wide range of topics that will need to be consulted. Strategies that can be used to manage the desk review include:

- Create a simple tracking document, listing, for example, the main title of the law, the topic, the detailed citation, whether the law is national or subnational, when it was passed and when it became effective, and the government entity responsible for its implementation. The categories of laws to be reviewed should be agreed upon in advance to allow comparison among government sectors involved in road safety.
- Organize a small brainstorming session or consult individuals and institutions to help identify laws or regulations relating to road safety, by asking whether there are laws or regulations on:
    - each of the risk factors–speed, drink–driving and use of motorcycle helmets, seat-belts and child restraints;
    - helmet standards;
    - post-crash care;
    - vehicle manufacture standards.

Topics related to road safety that would be expected to be addressed in laws or regulations include:

- safe behaviour with regard to speed, drink–driving and use of seat-belts, child restraints and motorcycle helmets;

Chapter 2 Assessing and improving laws and regulations

- the vehicle and the driver, including driver licensing, vehicle registration and vehicle manufacture standards;
- post-crash care, including training and licensing of first responders, facility licensing standards, legal protection to people who give reasonable assistance to people who are injured, ill, in peril or otherwise incapacitated ('good Samaritan' laws), ambulance vehicle standards and emergency care standards;
- data collection and management, such as crash reporting requirements and data-sharing among relevant institutions;
- infrastructure, such as transport audits, road signage and signals;
- victims' rights and patients' privacy rights.

This list includes areas that are not specifically addressed in this manual but which, as part of the assessment exercise, can be highlighted for future action.

- Involve people in related sectors, such as health, transport, interior and justice.
- Set priorities for review by relevance, for example, by starting with national legislation on well-documented risk factors for fatalities or injuries and then addressing time frames and national priorities.
- Conduct a rapid assessment of laws in other countries in the region or of subnational laws and regulations in order to harmonize laws or regulations regionally or nationally, by asking:
  - Is there a law or regulation addressing the risk factor?
  - Does it establish a mandate or limit, such as a blood alcohol concentration standard, helmet-wearing for all riders, or seat-belt wearing for all occupants?
  - Does it address enforcement (e.g. primary enforcement), and are the methods the same subnationally or regionally?
  - Does it include penalties, and are the penalty types the same subnationally or regionally?
  - What are the challenges to its implementation?
  - What have the outcomes been (especially if the law is relatively new)?

Information from the *Global status report on road safety 2013 (3)* can help in answering some of these questions. A comparison of the status of legislation in the 2009 and 2013 reports indicates which countries have passed new laws or upgraded existing laws. *(3, 4)*

2.3 Assessing the gaps in laws and regulations

Assessing gaps in legislation will ensure that any proposed changes are correctly targeted. The answers to the following questions can identify gaps in current legislation:

- Are there inconsistent or conflicting provisions?
- Are there too many exclusions and exceptions?
- Do the laws cover all risk factors?
- Do the problems identified compromise enforcement?
- Can the provisions be implemented and enforced?
- Does the law contribute to achieving the purpose for which it was enacted?

The answers to these questions will require a review of available information. Unfortunately, in many low-and middle-income countries, the information used for decision-making is sometimes difficult to obtain. In order for governments to assess the problems, policies and institutional settings for road safety, good data are however necessary *(5)*. The WHO publication, *Data systems: a road safety manual for decision-makers and practitioners (6)* describes a systematic approach for collecting, analysing and interpreting data for making decisions for effective road safety management. The absence of a comprehensive or reliable data system impedes understanding of the true nature of a problem, which has important implications for the solutions proposed to address the problem.

Comprehensive, reliable data are also necessary to evaluate the impact of changes. While most countries have legislation on risk factors such as speed, seat-belt wearing, helmet-wearing, drink–driving and child restraints, few have systems in place to monitor their effectiveness at national level, making it difficult to monitor and evaluate changes *(3)*.

Box 2.2 illustrates how a review of a law on wearing seat-belts in Turkey exposed exclusions that resulted in low rates of compliance. Box 2.3 shows how analysis of data on helmet-wearing rates in Cambodia resulted in the stepwise improvement to the motorcycle helmet-wearing law.

Some gaps may already be known, and attempts (perhaps unsuccessful) may have been made to rectify them. For example, the need for a law on child restraint was identified in Egypt some years ago, but the barrier was the cost *(7)*. The market availability of child restraints can also be a limiting factor. The status of a previously identified gap or issue may help in setting priorities and planning future action. For example:

- If a new law, regulation or amendment has already been drafted, much of the work on understanding the issue may have already been done; thus, the focus could turn to finding an opportunity to move the draft to the next step.
- If a working group or other body has been charged with conducting a review and making recommendations on laws and regulations, the focus could be on finding out what has been done and determining the next steps, such as making sure the recommendations are being considered and action is being taken by decision-makers.
- If a policy has been defined but has not moved to the legislative or regulatory phase, the focus could be on working with nongovernmental organizations to advocate for legislative change.

For some laws and regulations, expert input may be needed to define the problem; examples include motorcycle helmet specifications, vehicle inspection, blood alcohol testing, certain speed control requirements, ambulance standards, first responder training and certification requirements. Reliance on the technical expertise of either private or public sector bodies ensures accurate interpretation of the requirements and will make sure that those requirements are consistent with the best available evidence and standards.

Once the technical standards have been identified, laws or regulations must be evaluated to determine whether they prevent circumvention of the standard or whether new provisions are required to prevent such circumvention. In the case of motorcycle helmets, additional provisions might be needed to cover:

- mandating the inclusion of instructions for the proper care and fit of helmets and product labelling requirements (e.g. packaging laws and regulations);
- prohibiting the sale of noncompliant helmets and including penalties for violations and how the penalties will be imposed (e.g. sales inspections and seizures);
- prohibiting illegal imports and imposing penalties for importation of helmets that do not meet the country's recognized standards (e.g. import and customs laws and regulations);
- prohibiting tampering with helmets or product labels (de-specification) and imposing penalties (e.g. criminal and consumer protection laws and regulations and systems for reporting).

Countries that adopt helmet standards for the first time may find it difficult to put in place all laws, regulations and monitoring and enforcement systems at the same time. All legal measures should, however, be included in a long-term plan for comprehensive helmet-wearing laws and regulations.

Public perceptions about existing laws and regulations can shed light on whether and how they should be strengthened. Lack of clarity, misinterpretation or loopholes may become apparent when stakeholders and the public are engaged through focus groups, interviews or observational studies and surveys of knowledge, attitudes and practice. For example, studies that show that people generally do not strap

Box 2.2 Data help in making a case for change at local level

Step 1. Identify the problem

Seat-belt use first became mandatory in Turkey in 1986 under Article 78 of the Highway Traffic law. The law was phased-in for drivers and front-seat passengers in January 1992 and for all back-seat passengers in November 1995. Despite these legal provisions, seat-belt wearing rates remained low.

Step 2. Determine the nature of the problem

A number of causes were identified, including gaps in the law, lack of enforcement and poor public perception of the benefits of seat-belt wearing. In particular:

Broad exceptions continued to impede the effectiveness of the law on mandatory seat-belt wearing. The exceptions included military vehicles, emergency vehicles and certain classes of commercial vehicles and minibuses.

Although seat-belt wearing rates continued to be low, few fines were collected for not wearing a seat-belt especially after 2009. Between 2009 and 2010, seat-belt-related fines declined by 24%), raising concern about enforcement.

Studies of knowledge, attitudes and practice suggested that the general public did not understand the safety benefits of seat-belts. The reasons for noncompliance included discomfort, a perception that they were not necessary and inconvenience for pregnant women.

Step 3. Understand the consequences of the problem

A study by the Presidency of Traffic Training and Research in 2009 showed low rates of seat-belt wearing ; for example, rates as low as 17% were recorded on intra-city roads in Afyon.

Outcome of the assessment

The analysis resulted in two broad conclusions: a need for legislative changes to close the broad loopholes and non-legislative solutions including public education about the benefits of seat-belt wearing (through social marketing) and strengthened enforcement (through police training). Turkey's programme for aligning its laws and regulations with those of the European Union (2007–2013) includes amending highway traffic regulations with respect to the use of seat-belts. While awaiting legislative change at national level, the governor of Afyon issued a circular in March 2012 requiring all Government workers to wear seat-belts and be subject to enforcement. The seat-belt wearing rate rose from 17% to 50% after the circular was issued in Afyon. A similar circular was issued in Ankara in August 2012 following Afyon's success.

Source: reference *(8)*.

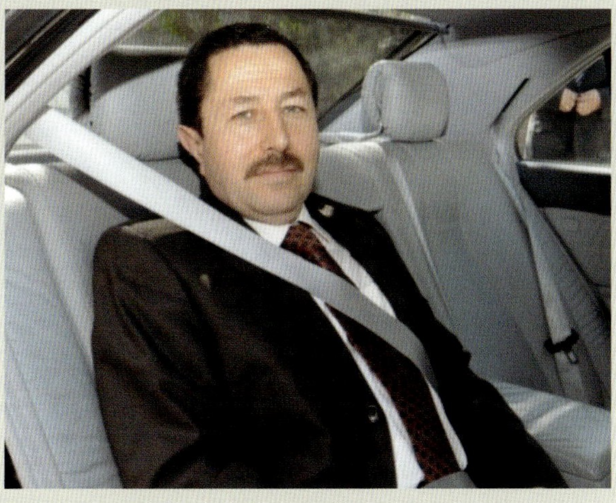

Copyright: Afyonkarahisar Governor - Irfan Balkanlioglu (c) Afyon provincial security directorate, 2012.

Box 2.3 Motorcycle helmet law in Cambodia

High injury and fatality rates among motorcyclists prompts further investigation of helmet-wearing rates

In 2004, a national database was established to provide the Government of Cambodia and other stakeholders with accurate, comprehensive information on road traffic crashes and their victims. The information system collects data from health facilities and traffic police in all of the country's 24 municipalities and provinces, and analyses and disseminates it for planning, implementing and evaluating appropriate policy and programme responses. Data from this system are complemented by primary data collection (such as observational studies on risk factors). Together, these data guide policy and action for reducing road traffic injuries in Cambodia.

Data from the system showed that the number of fatalities among motorcyclists increased by 61% between 2005 and 2010, after huge increases in levels of motorization. In 2008, motorcycles accounted for 75% of all motorized vehicles in Cambodia, and about 70% of all 1600 road traffic-related deaths were among motorcyclists (nearly half of whom suffered head trauma).

A decrease in helmet-wearing, particularly at night, indicated a need for legislation change or behaviour modification

Further analysis of data from the information system showed that almost half of the fatalities occurred between 16:00 and 22:00, particularly in the capital, Phnom Penh, where the number of motorcycle casualties increased fourfold between 2006 and 2008 and the percentage of fatalities was higher than in the rest of the country. Observational data showed that the helmet-wearing rate was low: about 47% of motorcycle drivers wore helmets in the daytime but only 36% of riders wore them during the evening.

A legislative measure to address this issue was introduced in 2007, with a law mandating the use of motorcycle helmets, signed by the King. Enforcement of the law began in January 2009, primarily in Phnom Penh at night, with the support of traffic police in setting up check-points. These night-time checkpoints simultaneously addressed the problem of drink–driving. At the same time, observational data were collected for monitoring and evaluating helmet-wearing rates.

Preliminary results suggest increased rates of helmet-wearing following introduction of the new law

Data collected in three provinces suggest that this legislative measure and its enforcement have increased the helmet-wearing rate and reduced the number of head injuries. Although the results of continual observation at three sites, where the law was actively enforced over a period of 5 months during 2010, showed an increase in helmet-wearing rates among drivers, the rates among passengers remained remained extremely low, partly because the legislation did not cover use of helmets by passengers.

In 2011, a multisectoral group proposed an amendment to the national road safety legislation to make passenger helmet-wearing mandatory. The proposed revision also includes a fivefold increase in the penalty associated with non-use of a helmet by all motorcycle users. In early 2012, the amendment was submitted for approval to the Council of Ministers, who will send it to the National Assembly, the Senate and ultimately the King. Social marketing will be used to support the legislative amendment by increasing awareness of the dangers of non-use of helmets by motorcyclists, including passengers.

Improvements in motorcycle helmet legislation continues

The next steps will include creating and implementing a national motorcycle helmet standard to ensure that all helmets sold provide a minimum level of protection.

helmets on correctly might indicate that the definition of 'helmet-wearing' should include 'strapping', as has been done in India and Viet Nam for example, combined with education on proper helmet-wearing.

Clarity in the text of a law is important, taking into account the language in which the law is written, cultural norms and legal or regulatory drafting standards (see Box 2.4).

Input from stakeholders and the public concerning their understanding or perception of laws can point to areas that require clarification. Nevertheless, changing laws or regulations can be time-consuming, and public education through mass media campaigns can resolve some of the confusion. It is important to assess whether improving compliance will best be done by a legislative or regulatory change or whether public education will suffice.

2.4 Improving the comprehensiveness of laws and regulations

The comprehensiveness of current road safety laws and regulations should be assessed to determine whether they:

- address all the important elements of each risk factor on the basis of the best available evidence;
- include enforcement mechanisms and resources;
- establish consequences for noncompliance.

Comprehensive legislation and regulation is important for the effectiveness of road safety measures.

2.4.1 Ensure that laws and regulations are based on evidence

Laws and regulations should establish mandatory requirements that are based on the best available evidence. In order to be comprehensive, a law or regulation should contain those elements that have been proven to shown scientifically to effect change. For example, graduated driving licensing laws are based on the premise that novice drivers should begin driving under relatively safe, low-risk conditions and be introduced gradually to more complex, higher-risk driving conditions *(9)*. The elements of law required to create 'low-risk' conditions must be consistent with the evidence in order to achieve the desired results; these elements might include restrictions on alcohol, limiting driving at night or with many peer passengers when first licenced, and limiting driving without supervision *(10, 11)*. Similarly, laws for transporting children in vehicles must specify the age, height and weight and the type of restraint to which the law or regulation applies *(12)*. Table 2.2 rates various interventions in terms of their effectiveness in preventing road traffic injuries among children that can be used to set national laws and regulations.

Basing laws and regulations on evidence is important for many reasons. Evidence provides a sound basis for moving an issue on

Box 2.4 Ensuring clarity in legal text

THE FOLLOWING ARE TWO EXAMPLES of how laws can be misinterpreted:

The statement, 'All individuals riding a motorcycle should wear a helmet' may not be interpreted as mandatory, particularly if there are no provisions for fines, enforcement or if enforcement is inconsistent. Conversely, *'All individuals riding a motorcycle must wear a helmet'* gives a clear mandate–enforcement and penalties notwithstanding–although these are necessary in order for the law or regulation to be considered comprehensive.

The statement, 'Not wearing a helmet may result in a penalty of 100–200 shillings' does not clearly set the fine, and may give officers too much leeway to determine the fine or may provide an opportunity for abuse by enforcement officers. *'All individuals not wearing a helmet will be fined 100 shillings'* is a clearer statement of the law and of expectations regarding penalties.

to the national legislative agenda, indicates alternative solutions to the problem and links the law to benefits for the general public, which is an important consideration when advocating for change.

A number of sources of evidence can be used. Studies conducted in various settings improve understanding of, for example, the link between car impact speed and fatality risk. Such information is helpful for determining speed limits on highways and in built-up areas, blood alcohol limits for novices, restraint use for older children and the effectiveness of speed cameras for enforcing speed limits.

In some areas, more research is required to determine the most effective intervention to promulgate as law. For example, more research is needed on sources of driver distraction, such as devices used while driving (e.g. handheld or wireless mobile phones and iPods). Laws banning the use of such devices while driving vary *(13)*.

When the evidence is not available or is inconclusive, a decision on whether to propose legislative change might be based on consideration of the evolution of road safety in the country and how it has been integrated into its laws and regulations. A country that has achieved significant reductions in injuries and fatalities might implement measures to achieve zero fatalities. Table 2.3 shows the evolution of the focus of road safety interventions as new results became available. Another approach might be to conduct a pilot study of a proposed measure and to use local data on its impact on road traffic injuries and fatalities to advocate for a national law.

2.4.2 Ensure that laws and regulations include appropriate provisions for enforcement

Laws and regulations should set out clear enforcement provisions, as consistent, sustained

Table 2.2 Strategies to prevent road traffic injuries among children

Strategy	Effective	Promising	Insuficient evidence	Ineffective	Harmful
Introducing (and enforcing) laws on minimum drinking age	✔				
Setting (and enforcing) lower blood alcohol limits for novice drivers and zero tolerance for offenders	✔				
Using appropriate child restraints and seat belts	✔				
Wearing motorcycle and bicycle helmets	✔				
Reducing speed around schools, residential areas and play areas	✔				
Separating different types of road user	✔				
Introducing (and enforcing) daytime running lights for motorcycles	✔				
Introducing a graduated driver licensing system	✔				
Implementing designated driver programmes			✔		
Increasing the visibility of pedestrians			✔		
Introducing instruction in schools on the dangers of drink–driving			✔		
Conducting school-based driver education				✔	
Seating infants and children in a place with an air bag					✔
Licensing novice adolescent drivers					✔

Source: Reference *(14)*

Table 2.3 Evolution of approaches to road safety, 1950s to present-day

Period	Phase	Description
Focus on driver interventions		
1950s–1960s	Phase 1	Emphasis on interventions to change behaviour, including laws and penalties
Focus on system interventions		
1970s–1980s	Phase 2	A systematic framework for road safety developed by William Haddon in 1970 to examine the role of personal attributes, vector or agent attributes, and environmental attributes (Haddon matrix) before, after and during crashes
		System-wide approach to road safety, including institutions, vehicles and infrastructure
Early 1990s	Phase 3	Targeting of institutional leadership and interventions by monitoring and evaluation
		Emphasis on intergovernmental and multisectoral coordination
		Setting target hierarchies
Late 1990s	Phase 4	Long-term elimination of serious crash-related injuries and fatalities
		Rethinking of interventions and institutional arrangements to reach an ambitious goal; examples include the Dutch 'sustainable safety' and Sweden's 'vision zero', and 'safe systems' approaches which have influenced initiatives in Australia, Denmark, Finland, Norway and Switzerland
Post 2000s	Current/ongoing	Continued emphasis on system-wide interventions, multisectoral responsibility, ambitious targets, effective institutional management and evidence-based interventions
		Investigation of innovative solutions

Source: *reference (15).*

enforcement of laws or regulations is critical to the effectiveness of interventions (Table 2.4). Enforcement may be inadequate because of a variety of social, economic, capacity, political and other factors. One way to mitigate this problem is ensure that the law or regulation clearly states how enforcement will be done and defines who is responsible for enforcement.

While a law may be enforced without a specific provision, an indication of how the law will be enforced and by whom can clarify the obligations of governmental entities, empower officials to perform their duties and show that funding is required for enforcement. In addition, clear enforcement provisions provide the basis for collecting evidence. For example, a law mandating blood alcohol testing at hospitals after serious or fatal crashes can generate useful data on alcohol-related crashes. Examples of how laws address enforcement of blood alcohol limits include the following:

- India's Motor Vehicle Act authorizes police officers to conduct a breath test if they have reasonable cause to suspect that an individual is violating drinking and driving laws.

Table 2.4 Effectiveness of enforcement measures relating to road traffic crashes

Enforcement measure	Percentage change in number of road traffic-related injuries and fatalities[a]		
	Fatal crashes	Injury crashes	All
Stationary speed enforcement	– 14 (–20; –8)	–6 (–9; –4)	
Patrolling	–4 (–32; +36)	–16 (–20; –12)	
Reduction of blood alcohol limit	–8(–12; –4)	–4 (–5; –3)	
Random breath testing[b]	–76 ... –16	–28...–10	
Drink–driving enforcement	–9 (–11; –6)	–7 (–8; –6)	
Seat belt enforcement	–6(–21; +14)	–8 (–18; +4)	
Speed cameras		–17 (–19; –16)	–19 (–20; –18)
Cameras at red lights		–12	–11 (–18; –3)
Fines, withdrawal of driving licence, imprisonment (total effect)			–10 (–11; –9)
Warning letters			–15 (–18; –13)
Demerit point system			–5 (–10; 0)
Driving licence suspension			–17 (–19; –16)

[a] Entries represent most likely effect and 95% confidence interval.

[b] Random breath testing results are from Peek-Asa *(16)* and are based on the number of victims not crashes; most likely effect not available; only ranges at 95% confidence interval provided.

Sources: adapted references *(17, 18)*.

In addition, in the case of a crash, police officers have the authority to administer a breath test if they have reasonable cause to believe that the person who was driving the motor vehicle at the time of the crash had alcohol in his or her blood or was driving under the influence of other specified drugs. If the driver is hospitalized after a crash, however, the attending physician must be notified and must approve the test before a police officer conducts it. The physician can object to testing on the grounds that its provision or the requirement to provide it would be prejudicial to the proper care or treatment of the patient *(2)*.

- In the United States, while drivers can be stopped randomly at 'sobriety check-points', a blood alcohol test cannot be administered unless there is suspicion of alcohol use. In some states, however, refusal to undergo a blood alcohol test is treated as a violation and can result in administrative penalties. In Maryland, if a person holding a state licence refuses to take a blood alcohol test, the police officer can confiscate the driver's licence, issue a temporary paper licence and prepare a case for the Maryland Motor Vehicles Administration. If the driver is a commercial vehicle operator, the Administration will suspend or disqualify his or her driving privileges *(19)*.

- Police in Australia can conduct random breath tests on any driver or motorcycle rider at any time without having identified a problem. Interventions can include readily identifiable 'booze buses', in which drivers are taken for further blood testing if a blood alcohol test is positive. In some states, all police vehicles are equipped with breathalysers to ensure that a breath test can be conducted if an incident occurs *(16)*.

- Regulations in China allow use of a detecting device as a prerequisite for administering a breathalyser.

Box 2.5 Malaysia's stepped approach to implementing a passenger seat-belt law

MALAYSIA USED A 6-MONTH PHASED APPROACH to implement its passenger seat-belt law once it was passed, which started with a series of safety promotion campaigns, followed by awareness-raising activities and finally enforcement. The safety promotion strategy included a social marketing campaign and education about rear seat-belt safety and the information phasing-in requirements for older vehicles. For example, owners of cars registered after 1995 without belt mountings were given a 3-year grace period to retrofit the car with rear seat-belts. Community programmes to create awareness among Malaysians included participation by high-level entities, such as the Road Safety Department, the Royal Malaysia Police and the Road Transport Department to promote the use of rear seat-belts. During the advocacy period, police enforcement included stern advice and warnings about the penalties of noncompliance. Full implementation of the law took effect on 1 January 2009.

Source: references *(20, 21)*.

Another option is staged enforcement of a law over time, to allow the public to integrate the law into their daily lives and foster community policing. For example, police can issue warnings and provide education before beginning to impose sanctions (Box 2.5). This option could also be used in the case of a law requiring for example mandatory helmet-wearing when helmet standards have not yet been put in place.

2.4.3 Ensure that laws and regulations include appropriate penalties

Penalties should be appropriate and based on current knowledge of their effectiveness. A variety of penalties have been used to change road user behaviour, including warnings, financial penalties (fixed or based on degree of offence), demerit point systems, licence suspension, vehicle impoundment and imprisonment. In some cases, driver insurance rates are tied to the record of driving violations, resulting in higher premium rates as an additional form of financial penalty. Penalties are sometimes combined, such as both financial penalties and demerit points for speeding violations. Driver improvement programmes may be mandated or offered as an alternative to financial penalties for severe or repeat offenders. Research suggests that targeted programmes can reduce both recidivism and court costs *(22, 23)*.

Penalties should be appropriate as severity alone does not ensure the effectiveness of penalties *(24)*.

For example:

- Variable fines, such as those based on a proportion of the income of the offender, ensure that road users are equally affected financially for the same traffic offence.
- Substantial increases in fines for relatively minor offences may undermine other aspects of the criminal justice system; therefore, fines should be set in relation to the amount of other fines in the criminal justice system.
- Fines that are too low may send the message to drivers that illegal driving behaviour is affordable *(25)*.

Although the effectiveness of certain types of penalties on violations of road safety laws has been the subject of many studies, it is often difficult to isolate the effect of sanctions because they are usually combined with other measures, and the results have not been consistent. Nevertheless, some studies indicate the effectiveness of certain sanctions on certain types of violations under certain conditions (Table 2.5). The costs of administering sanctions should also be taken into account, as well as the likelihood that the sanction will be consistently administered; otherwise, its effectiveness is reduced. Matching the amount of the fine to the consumer price index or another suitable index can prevent fines from appearing to be too low over time.

Table 2.5 Effectiveness of penalties for driving violations

Penalty type	Description	Effectiveness
Fixed	Includes fines administered on the scene, usually for common violations such as speeding, disregarding road signs, not stopping at red lights, with no need for court appearance.	May reduce violations, but the results of studies are inconsistent. Increases the use of seat-belts. No demonstrable effect on speeding.
Administrative license suspension	Police can suspend the licence of a driver who does not pass a blood alcohol test, without a court appearance.	Reduces the number of fatal crashes, with a greater effect in alcohol-related fatal crashes. Laws requiring a court appearance appear to be less effective than administrative licence suspension. Effective only among drivers whose licence has already been suspended and only during the time the licence was suspended.
Demerit point system	Drivers are assessed on a point system for serious violations or crashes and receive a sanction once a critical threshold has been reached. Sanctions can include warning letters, mandatory driver improvement courses or licence suspension.	Does not reduce crashes, although components of such systems may do so. Courses and warning letters reduced crashes by around 10%. Drivers who accumulate enough points and risk licence suspension (notified via warning letters) become more cautious. As the effectiveness of warning letters depends on their content, the results are not consistent. Driver improvement courses reduced crashes involving young drivers.
Vehicle impoundment	Police can administratively confiscate the violator's vehicle (even if he or she is not the owner) for offences such as an illegal blood alcohol concentration or driving without a valid licence. Impounded vehicles can be returned after the impoundment period against payment of a fee. When the impounded vehicle belongs to someone other than the violator, the vehicle can be reinstated to the owner under certain conditions. As alternatives, the licence plate may be seized, a sticker may be attached to the licence plate or the vehicle registration may be withdrawn.	For drivers convicted of driving under the influence of alcohol, vehicle impoundment has a greater, longer-lasting effect than licence suspension, even if there is only a threat of impoundment (e.g. in jurisdictions where driving with a suspended licence can result in vehicle impoundment). The deterrent effect may be due to drivers wanting to avoid further penalties or problems with people from whom they borrow vehicles, as well as reduced access to vehicles, as drivers may find it more difficult to borrow vehicles and not all impounded vehicles are retrieved by the owner.
Imprisonment	Some road traffic offences are criminalized in certain countries, such as those resulting in a fatality.	In jurisdictions where drink–driving is criminalized, imprisonment has been found to be effective, in particular when combined with a court-administered programme (generally including sanctions, treatment and monitoring). Otherwise, imprisonment has not been found to reduce crashes involving drink–driving

Source: adapted from reference *(26)*.

2.5 References

1. Passmore J et al. The formulation and implementation of a national helmet law: a case study for Viet Nam. *Bulletin of the World Health Organization,* 2010, 88:783–787.

2. *Report of the Expert Committee: Review of the Motor Vehicles Act, 1988, submitted to Ministry of Roads Transport and Highways.* New Delhi, Ministry of Road Transport and Highways, 2011 (http://morth.nic.in/index.asp, accessed 10 January 2013).

3. *Global status report on road safety* 2013: supporting a decade of action. Geneva, World Health Organization, 2013.

4. *Global status report on road safety: time for action.* Geneva, World Health Organization, 2009.

5. Peden M et al., eds. *World report on road traffic injury prevention.* Geneva, World Health Organization, 2004.

6. *Data systems: a road safety manual for decision-makers and practitioners.* Geneva, World Health Organization, 2010.

7. *The EU-Twinning expertise for enhancing road safety in Egypt: Germany, Austria, Egypt 2008–2011 (Twinning Project No. EG08/AA/TP13)* (http://www.svpt.uni-wuppertal.de/fileadmin/bauing/svpt/Publikationen/The_Twinning_Expertise_for_Enhancing_Road_Safety_in_Egypt_01.pdf, accessed 9 January 2013).

8. Öztürk EA. *Road safety in 10 countries: highway traffic legislation in Turkey. Final report.* Ankara, World Health Organization Country Office, 2011.

9. Hartling L et al. Graduated driver licensing for reducing motor vehicle crashes among young drivers. *Cochrane Database of Systematic Reviews,* 2009, Issue 1.

10. *National road safety strategy 2011–2020.* Canberra, Australian Transport Council, 2010 (http://www.atcouncil.gov.au/documents/files/NRSS_2011_2020_15Aug11.pdf, accessed 10 January 2013).

11. Insurance Institute for Highway Safety. *Young driver licensing systems in the US.* Arlington, VA, Highway Loss Data Institute, 2011 (http://www.iihs.org/laws/graduatedLicenceIntro.aspx, accessed 9 January 2013).

12. Dellinger A et al. Interventions to prevent motor vehicle injuries. In: Doll LS et al., eds. *Handbook of injury and violence prevention.* New York, Springer, 2007:55–79.

13. *Mobile phone use: a growing problem of driver distraction.* Geneva, World Health Organization, 2011

14. Peden M et al., eds. *World report on child injury prevention.* Geneva, World Health Organization, 2008.

15. *Towards zero: ambitious road safety targets and the safe systems approach.* Paris, Organisation for Economic Co-operation and Development, International Transport Forum, 2008.

16. Peek-Asa C. The effect of random alcohol screening in reducing motor vehicle crash injuries. *American Journal of Preventive Medicine,* 1999, 16(1S):57–67.

17. Elvik R, Vaa T. *The handbook of road safety measures.* Amsterdam, Elsevier, 2004.

18. *Summary and publication of best practices in road safety in the Member States. Thematic report: enforcement.* Luxembourg, European Commission, 2007 (http://ec.europa.eu/transport/roadsafety_library/publications/supreme_f6_thematic_report_enforcement.pdf, accessed 10 January 2013).

19. Department of Transportation. *Alcohol test failure or refusal.* Baltimore, MD, Motor Vehicles Administration, 2011 (http://www.mva.maryland.gov/About-MVA/INFO/26100/26100-50T.htm, accessed 9 January 2013).

20. *Research report. Phase 1: Achievements of First 3-Month Advocacy Program. Rear seatbelt use: Public awareness and practice.* Malaysia, Malaysia Institute of Road Safety Research, 2008 (http://miros.gov.my/web/guest/reports, accessed 11 January 2013).

21. [Anonymous]. Enforcement of rear seat-belt from Jan 1. *The Malaysian Insider,* 7 June 2008 (http://www.themalaysianinsider.com/malaysia/article/Enforcement-of-rear-seat-belt-from-Jan-1, accessed 11 January 2013).

22. af Wahlberg AE. Re-education of young driving offenders: effects on recorded offences and self-reported collisions. *Transportation Research*, Part F, 2011, 14:291–299.

23. Voas RB et al. Towards a national model for managing impaired driving offenders. *Addiction*, 2011, 106:1221–1227.

24. Mohan D. *Analysis of penalties for traffic violations: magnitude and effectiveness, submitted to the Committee to Review Motor Vehicles Act 1988*. New Delhi, Transportation Research and Injury Prevention Programme, Indian Institute of Technology, 2009.

25. Zaal D. *Traffic law enforcement: a review of the literature*. Melbourne, Monash University Accident Research Centre, 1994 (Report #53) (http://www.monash.edu.au/miri/research/reports/muarc053.html, accessed 10 January 2013).

26. Elvik R et al. *The handbook of road safety measures*. New York, Emerald Publishing, *2009*.

Chapter 3

Practice and resources

Chapter 03 Practice and resources

3.1 Improving the comprehensiveness of laws relating to specific risk factors

The five main risk factors are: speeding, drink–driving, not using motorcycle helmets, seat-belts and child restraints. A process similar to that described below can be used to assess the comprehensiveness of laws relevant to these risk factors and for pedestrian safety, safe road infrastructure and vehicle design, for example. For each of the five main risk factors, the following are given in this chapter:

- *Problem statement*: to indicate why the topic should be addressed in a law or regulation. The statement does not reiterate evidence on the risk factor, which is covered in published manuals.
- *Global status of legislation*: to indicate gaps in legislation from a global perspective, highlighting the need for action. This section does not provide a comparative analysis of national legislation but shows what is still required.
- *Resources for evidence-based laws and regulation* to summarize the latest recommendations for mitigating the impact of the risk factor, in terms of setting standards and limits in laws and regulations, based on the best available scientific evidence. Research findings from selected countries are summarized, when available. Both the WHO 2013 *Global status report on road safety (1)* and the United Nations Economic Commission for Europe (UNECE) *Consolidated Resolution on Road Traffic (2)* give recommendations on legislation. WHO and partners have also published a series of practical guides to help decision-makers and practitioners implement, enforce and evaluate programmes on the five main risk factors *(3-6)* and develop appropriate data systems *(7)*. Recommendations should be relevant to the national context and reflect the level at which the best results in reducing fatalities and serious injuries can be achieved.
- *Enforcement and other regulatory measures*: to indicate other potential regulatory measures for addressing the risk factor.
- *A Checklist:* the sample checklist, which can be adapted to conduct the desk audit and identify gaps. With research and expert input, similar checklists can be prepared for other topics, such as pedestrian safety, road infrastructure and vehicle design. Broadly speaking, the key questions to ask when preparing a checklist include:
    - What is the evidence-based standard for the measure being considered?
    - Are there national or internationally recognized standards (for example, vehicle safety standards)?
    - Which enforcement mechanisms and penalties have been found to be the most effective in, for example, systematic reviews, the 'grey' literature and country case studies?

In addition, examples of current laws governing speed, drink–driving, motorcycle helmets and seat-belts are provided in the Annex. These are not intended as models but rather as reference points for drafting legislation.

3.1.1 Speed

Problem statement

Speed is a key risk factor in pedestrian injuries and fatalities. Research shows that an adult pedestrian has a 20% risk of dying if struck by a car travelling at 60 km/h, and an impact speed above 30 km/h increases the likelihood of severe injury or death *(8–10)*. Lowering speed limits backed by appropriate enforcement and education can help reduce serious injuries and fatalities.

Global status of legislation on speed limits

Lowering speed limits has been shown to reduce the risks for crashes and fatalities and also the severity of injuries and the number of fatalities. While safe speed thresholds vary by the type of road and road user, research on effective speed management has shown that the limit on urban roads should not exceed 50 km/h. Based on the 2013 *Global status report*, only half of the countries responding to the questionnaire implement an urban speed limit of less than or equal to 50 km/h and allow local authorities to reduce this where appropriate. Even in countries with lower speed limits, enforcement was often lacking or inadequate *(1)*.

Resources for evidence-based laws and regulations

The 2013 *Global status report on road safety (1)* recommends that countries set speed limits by taking into account vehicle type, the nature of the road, roadside activities and use by vulnerable groups. The UNECE *Consolidated resolution on road traffic (2)* gives recommendations on safe speed thresholds by type of road, thus focusing on the road function and hierarchy in determining the best applicable speed limit. The UNECE recommendations are:

- roads on which there are possible conflicts between cars and unprotected users: 30 km/h;
- intersections at which there are possible side-on conflicts between cars: 50 km/h;
- roads on which there are possible frontal conflicts between cars: 70 km/h;
- roads on which there is no likelihood of frontal or side-on conflicts between road users: ≥ 100 km/h.

The UNECE also recommends that speed limits be based on the type of road (urban roads, motorways, dual carriageways, other roads), type of vehicle (light, heavy), type of user (e.g. novice driver) and environmental conditions (such as rain, snow and fog). It also recommends that local conditions and emergency or temporary measures be taken into account, such as unexpected events affecting road safety *(2)*.

Enforcement and other regulatory measures

The 'safe system' approach to road safety ensures that, in a crash, the impact energy remains below the threshold likely to result in death or serious injury *(11)*. It goes beyond establishing speed limits, to managing interactions between the environment, infrastructure and physical vulnerability. Thus, speed limits are a complementary intervention to creating safer roads, roadsides and vehicles. The approach includes use of effective speed measurement devices to change behaviour and making both vehicles and roads safer to accommodate behavioural lapses in driving. In a safe system approach, laws and regulations could include:

- *Automatic speed measurement devices*: Speed cameras are effective in reducing road traffic injuries and fatalities in both rural and urban settings (see Box 3.1); however, there is little empirical evidence of the relative effectiveness of covert versus overt automatic speed cameras *(12)*.
- *Speed governors, (including mandatory use in commercial and other vehicle fleets:)* In Australia, vehicles with a gross mass of more than 12 tonnes and buses of more than 5 tonnes must be fitted with a speed limiter set to limit the maximum speed by acceleration to 100 km/h. There are also initiatives in Ontario and other provinces in Canada to mandate the use of speed limiters in heavy vehicles *(13)*.
- *Safer roads and roadsides:* Institution of 'traffic-calming' measures (e.g. traffic

Box 3.1 Effectiveness and cost benefits of fixed speed cameras in the United Kingdom

SPEED CAMERAS WERE FIRST used for enforcement in the United Kingdom in 1992, following a review of the road traffic law in 1988. As part of a national safety programme, the installation of fixed speed cameras was accelerated between 2001 and 2005. Speed was reduced by about 70% after installation of the fixed cameras, and actual vehicle speeds decreased by an average of 6%. Use of fixed cameras has been cited as a reason why the number of deaths on UK roads fell from about 5000 a year in the early 1990s to 1850 in 2010. At camera sites, there were 32% fewer fatalities and 42% fewer people injured per annum.

An association was found between a reduction in speed and a reduction in collisions resulting in personal injury. Safety cameras are funded from revenue raised from fines.

The cost of enforcement, including public education, is estimated to be about US$ 150 million, while the estimated cost saving accrued from fewer collisions is about US$ 410 million, giving an estimated benefit–cost ratio of 2.7.

Source: reference *(14)*.

Road traffic deaths in the UK

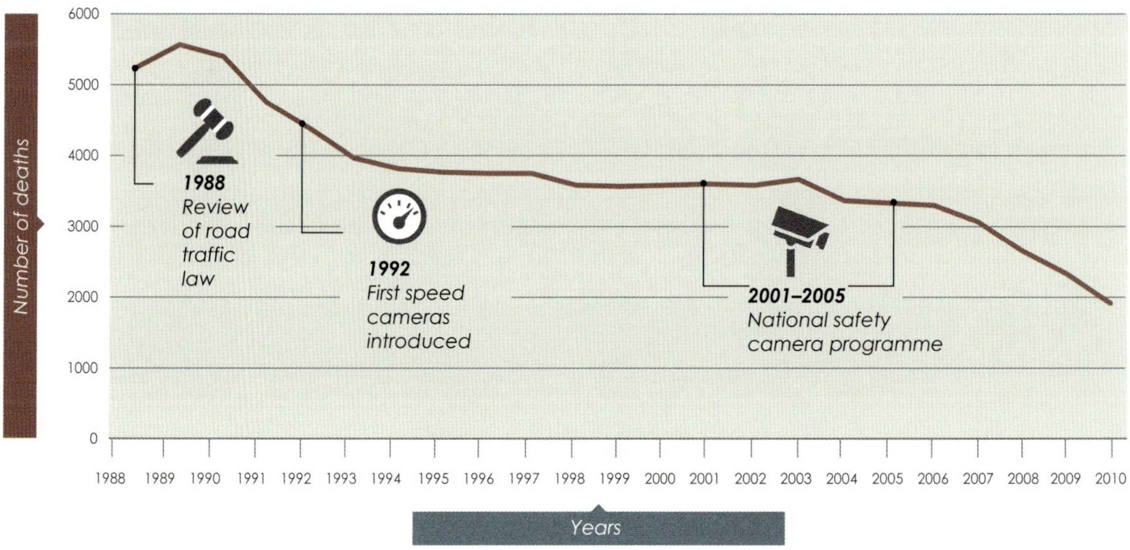

circles and rumple strips) can help reduce speeds. The adoption of minimum road safety audit requirements in construction or maintenance projects can help ensure that such measures are taken into consideration in designing roads. A checklist for assessing the comprehensiveness of speed legislation is contained in Table 3.1.

Table 3.1 Checklist for assessing the comprehensiveness of speed legislation

Does the content of current legislation address:

1 Maximum speed limits	Yes	No
Consistent with evidence and recommendations on safe speed (≤ 50 km/h on urban roads)		
Establishes speed limits by type of road		
Establishes speed limits by type of vehicle		
Establishes speed limits for all motorized vehicles		
Establishes speed limits by road hierarchy		
Use of radar detection		
Further reduction of speed limits by local authorities		
Provides narrowly construed exclusions or exceptions, such as for emergency vehicles		
2 Enforcement		
Provides notice requirements for certain enforcement activity, if applicable		
Specifies covert versus overt automatic speed limit enforcement		
Provides authority for enforcement		
3 Penalties		
Defines penalty (financial and demerit points) based on degree of severity of infraction above established limit.		
Provides specific financial penalties		
Includes provision for driver remediation		
Provides for licence suspension based on degree of severity of infraction above established limit		
Includes provisions pertaining to vehicle impoundment		
Specifies whether penalty includes criminal punishment, with reference to penal code if applicable		
4 Other speed management measures		
Includes highway design standards that specify recommended speed limits		
Includes road audit requirements		

3.1.2 Drink–driving

Problem statement

Impairment of reflexes by alcohol has serious consequences on the road. Drivers who have been drinking have a higher risk for being involved in a crash and a greater likelihood of resulting death or serious injury. They also put other road users at risk. The risk for a crash increases significantly at a blood alcohol concentration ≥ 0.04 g/dl *(15-19)* (see Figure 3.1).

The amount of alcohol in the blood is measured by testing a sample of blood or urine. It can also be estimated from the breath alcohol concentration with a device called a 'breathalyser'. As research has shown an accurate correspondence between the breath and the blood alcohol concentration, this is the mechanism used generally in the context of road safety. The use of breathalysers in law enforcement and the extent to which the results obtained with a breathalyser can be used as evidence for prosecution in drink–driving cases must, however, be described very clearly in laws and regulations in order to avoid setbacks in implementing drink–driving interventions.

Global status of legislation on drink–driving

A main finding in the 2013 *Global status report on road safety* is that the blood alcohol concentrations used to establish a legal definition of drink–driving vary from country to country. In less than half the countries with drink–driving laws the threshold blood alcohol concentration set at ≤ 0.05 g/dl, which is the recommended limit for the general population *(1)*.

Figure 3.1 Relative risk of driver involvement in road traffic crashes

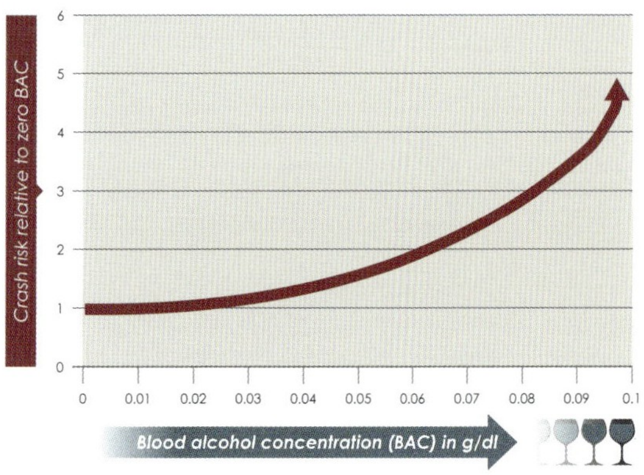

Source: reference *(19)*.

Resources for evidence-based laws and regulations

The 2013 *Global status report on road safety* recommends that laws on drink–driving should set the threshold blood alcohol concentration at ≤ 0.02 g/dl for young or novice drivers and at ≤ 0.05 g/dl for the population at large. A level of ≤ 0.02 g/dl for young or novice drivers reduces their risk for being involved in a crash by up to 24% *(1)*. The UNECE *(2)* also recommends that a blood alcohol level of ≤ 0.02 g/dl be established for drivers such as novices and commercial drivers and for drivers carrying dangerous goods.

Applying a blood alcohol level concentration limit of 0.02 g/dl or less for young and novice drivers is an effective way of reducing drink–driving related crashes for this group. An evaluation was conducted of six studies of fatalities and injuries among drivers in four Australian states (Queensland, Tasmania, Victoria and Western Australia) and three states in the United States (Maine, Maryland and Massachusetts) with blood alcohol limits ranging from 0 to 0.06 g/dl *(20)*. The participants were drivers aged 15–21 years who had been involved in serious or fatal crashes. The average reduction in fatalities in night-time crashes involving a single vehicle was 22% in jurisdictions with a zero blood alcohol restriction and 17% in jurisdictions with a 0.02 g/dl blood alcohol limit. In Australia, a zero blood alcohol concentration is recommended for these reasons, and all but one jurisdiction have adopted this restriction for probationary drivers *(21)*.

Enforcement and other regulatory measures

Primary policies to address drink–driving are based on deterrence and reducing the availability of alcohol. Other measures that should be covered in laws or regulations include:

- *Random breath testing:* Drivers are stopped randomly and given a breath test to determine whether their breath alcohol concentration is above the legal limit. Unlike at sobriety check-points, drivers who are stopped at random are required to take a breath test even if they are not suspected of any other offence, as in Sweden (see Box 3.2) *(22, 23)*.

- *Sobriety checkpoints:* Highly visible police officers systematically stop vehicles during the hours and days when there is a greater likelihood of drinking and give a breath test if the driver is suspected of drinking and driving. Depending on the country or jurisdiction (subnational), laws or regulations should clearly state the authority for administering a breath test. In Mexico, for example, police officers are prohibited by the Constitution from stopping a vehicle and administering a breath test unless the vehicle was stopped for another violation. Similarly, in some states of the USA, officers cannot administer a breath test without other evidence of intoxication because of constitutional protection against unreasonable searches and seizure *(24, 25)*. Some states in the USA have therefore adopted penalties as a disincentive for individuals to refuse testing, as recommended by the UNECE *Consolidated resolution on road traffic (2)*.
- *Administrative licence suspension or revocation:* These laws allow officers to seize the licence of anyone found to be driving with a blood alcohol concentration at or above the legal limit *(26)*. Such laws have been found to be effective in reducing alcohol-related crashes and fatalities, but they can be difficult to enforce, as some drivers continue to drive with a suspended licence *(23)*.
- *Minimum age for legal purchase or drinking of alcohol:* Establishing a minimum age for the purchase and public consumption of alcoholic beverages can reduce drinking and driving among young drivers, and is recommended by the UNECE *(2)*. The minimum age is usually between 16 and 21 years *(27)*. Increasing the legal age for drinking in Australia, Canada and the USA decreased the number of crashes due to drink–driving. Strict enforcement to prevent

Box 3.2 Effectiveness of random breath testing in Sweden

SINCE 1990, THE BLOOD ALCOHOL CONCENTRATION (BAC) limit in Sweden has been set at 0.02 g/dl. A criminal sanction of either a high fine or imprisonment is imposed on drivers recording a BAC in excess of 0.1 g/dl. The administrative sanction is suspension of the offender's driving licence for up to 3 years, depending on the blood alcohol level and recidivism. All offenders have to prove that they have a sober lifestyle before a new licence is issued. The law is enforced by random breath testing. It has been estimated that intoxicated drivers (with a BAC > 0.02 g/dl) cause 14% of collisions in which occupants sustain injuries. The risk that a drunk driver will be involved in a collision resulting in injuries is about 50 times higher than that of sober drivers. Strict random breath testing has reduced the proportion of injury-related collisions involving drunk drivers from 14% to 9%, in large part due to a reduction in exposure (fewer drunk drivers on the road) but also because of a change in the attitude of drivers to drinking and driving. In addition, alcohol interlocks have been fitted on fleet and personal vehicles since 1999.

Source: reference (22).

Evolution of drink-driving laws and regulations in Sweden, 1925-present-day

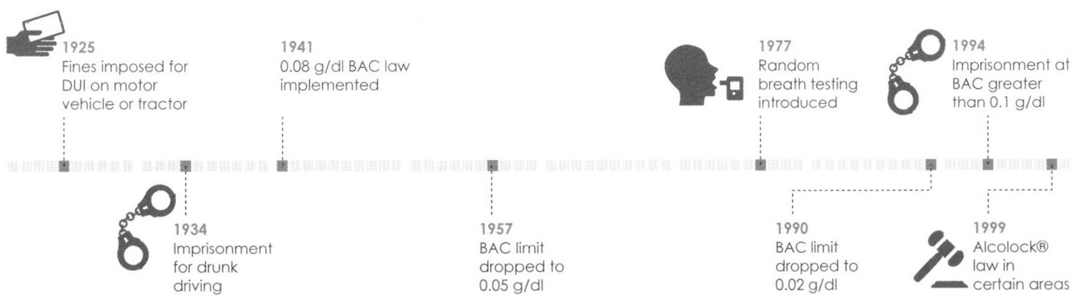

BAC, blood alcohol concentration;
DUI, driving under the influence of alcohol
Alcolock®, system that prevents a driver from starting a vehicle after recording a positive breath test

alcohol sales to underage people is critical to the effectiveness of such laws *(23)*.

- *Mandatory blood alcohol tests for all people involved in a crash:* Some countries require mandatory blood alcohol testing for anyone admitted to hospital after a crash. For example, in South Africa, a criminal procedure act authorizes collection of a blood or other specimen from individuals without their consent, and use of appropriate restraints if needed to collect such a sample *(28, 29)*. In India, a test may be administered only if there is reasonable cause to suspect the involvement of alcohol, and requires that notice be given to the attending physician, who can object if in their opinion the test would be prejudicial to the proper care or treatment of the individual *(30)*. In South Australia, a compulsory blood test is required for anyone who appears to be over 10 years of age who suffers an injury or fatality as a result of a car crash and is taken to hospital *(31)*. Mandatory testing can have the added benefit of improving data collection and reporting on alcohol-related crashes.

- *Alcohol ignition interlocks:* These devices lock the ignition of a vehicle and require that the driver first provide a breath sample (Box 3.3). The device must register a blood alcohol concentration that is lower than a pre-set threshold before the vehicle can start. The results of the breath test are logged into the system, and drivers are randomly retested while the vehicle is running to reduce circumvention of the device. These devices have been shown to be effective in reducing recidivism, at least while the device is in place *(32)*. In Sweden, alcohol interlocks were introduced in demonstration projects and then rolled out countrywide in October 2003; they are now installed in

Box 3.3 Legal framework for alcohol interlock programmes in the USA

IN THE USA, THE LEGAL AUTHORITY for alcohol interlock programmes differs from state to state. This has resulted a marked differences in the effectiveness and public health impact of such measures, as briefly outlined below:

- *Court authority:* Courts may impose the interlock as a sanctioning option under common law; however, this is largely discretionary, varying among judges and jurisdictions. Furthermore, under such programmes, court orders to install interlocks are often not processed by the motor vehicle or driver licensing authority. As a result, sanctions are not reflected on the licence records of an individual; consequently, officers who stop offenders do not check for an interlock. Some states have legislation that explicitly gives judges the authority to apply the sanction; however, this is still discretionary, tending to encourage judges to impose the sanction. Generally, mandatory laws requiring judges to impose the sanction have had limited impact, because of conflicts with strict licence suspension laws.

- *Administrative interlock programmes:* In these programmes, state laws specifically provide for the use of interlocks as a sanction for a drink–driving offence or for driving with a suspended licence resulting from a prior drink–driving offence. In these programmes, interlocks may be installed as an alternative to licence suspension (for the period during which a licence would otherwise have been suspended) or as a condition of licence reinstatement after suspension due to drink–driving. Some of the challenges to the effectiveness of alcohol interlocks as a prerequisite to reinstatement is that drivers might simply wait out the suspension period or not have their licence reinstated.

- *Administrative authority:* A state motor vehicle department might administer alcohol interlock programmes under their authority to regulate driver licensing in order to address drink–driving.

Source: reference *(33)*.

passenger cars, trucks, buses and taxis. The measure has gained wide acceptance by professional drivers, their employers and passengers *(34)*. Use of data obtained from these devices should be addressed in laws, particularly when they are used in the commercial sector. For example, in countries where exceeding the pre-set limit is a criminal offence and the test records a concentration above the limit, employers can either report the event or use the information to provide assistance to the worker. An important aspect is the legal authority governing the use of these devices (Box 3.3). Several other countries, such as Australia and Canada, have already introduced alcohol interlock programmes, and feasibility studies are being conducted in some countries of the European Union *(32)*. As several devices are available on the market, the price, accuracy, affordability, installation and relative ease of use should be considered when determining their cost–effectiveness *(35)*. A checklist for assessing the comprehensiveness of drink–driving legislation in contained in Table 3.2.

Table 3.2 Checklist for assessing the comprehensiveness of drink–driving legislation

Does the content of current legislation address:

	Yes	No
1 Blood alcohol concentration limits		
Imposes limits that are consistent with evidence and recommendations on drinking and driving (0.05 g/dl or below)		
Sets limits for both regular and novice or young drivers (BAC, 0.02 g/dl or below)		
2 Restrictions on availability of alcohol		
Specifies a minimum legal drinking age		
Imposes restrictions on sales of alcohol to underage people		
3 Enforcement		
Provides notice requirements for certain enforcement activity, if applicable		
Provides for enforcement by random breath testing or sobriety checkpoints		
Requires alcohol testing of everyone involved in a crash (in hospital or at the site of the crash)		
Establishes who has authority for enforcement		
Provides a mechanism to monitor the sale of alcohol to underage people in certain facilities		
4 Penalties		
Defines penalty (financial and demerit points) based on degree of severity of infraction above established BAC limit		
Provides specific financial penalties		
Includes provision for driver remediation		
Provides for licence suspension based on degree of severity of infraction above established limit		
Includes provisions pertaining to vehicle impoundment		
Specifies whether the penalty includes criminal punishment, with reference to the penal code if applicable		
5 Other drink–driving measures		
Authority for the use of alcohol ignition interlock programmes, including criteria for offenders		

3.1.3 Motorcycle helmets

Problem statement

Fatality rates among motorcyclists in low- and middle-income countries are typically higher than in high-income countries because of differences in levels of motorcycle ownership and use. In low- and middle-income countries they are used as family vehicles, delivery vehicles and taxis. In Africa, for example both, the demand for motorcycles and the number of motorcycles on the road have increased rapidly in the past decade (Box 3.4), partly because of the low cost of motorcycles and the inadequacy and inaccessibility of public transport *(36–38)*. There is therefore an urgent need for laws and standards on helmet use.

Box 3.4 Rapid motorization in Burkina Faso

IN 2000, BURKINA FASO'S FLEET of motorized vehicles (with four or more wheels) totalled 79 974; in 2007, the fleet had grown to nearly twice that number, i.e. to 158 981 vehicles. Most of this growth has been in private vehicles. The growth in the number of two-wheelers has been even more dramatic. In 1999, there were just over 80 000 two-wheelers with an engine capacity of 50 cc and above on Burkino Faso's roads; during the next 7 years, their number increased almost fourfold.

Source: reference *(36)*.

Growth of vehicle fleet, 1999–2006 (number of vehicles)

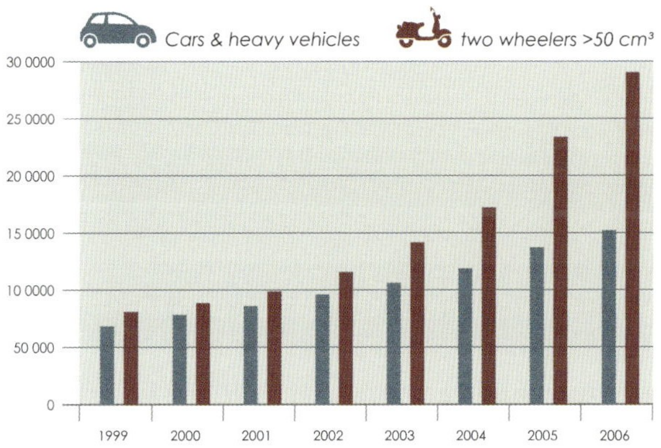

Global status of legislation on motorcycle helmets

Motorcycle helmets can reduce the risk of death by 42% and the risk of head injury by almost 70% *(39)*. Despite this evidence, onlyl less than half of all countries have a comprehensive helmet law covering all riders, all roads and all engine types, and apply a helmet standard *(1)*. Use of non-standard helmets is another problem: while helmet use is highly effective in reducing head injuries, the protective effect is substantially diminished if a non-standard helmet is used. According to the 2013 *Global status report on road safety*, however, only about half of countries require that helmets adhere to specific standards *(1)*. Box 3.5 describes the use of non-standard helmets in 10 low- and middle-income countries.

Resources for evidence-based laws and regulations

The *2013 Global status report on road safety* recommends laws mandating helmet-wearing for the drivers and passengers of all two- and three-wheeled motorized vehicles, of all engine types and on all road types. It also recommends enactment of laws that require helmets to meet national or international standards *(1)*.

Protective helmet standards are in place in the European region *(40)*. Some countries have set their own motorcycle helmet standards, taking into account evidence on their effectiveness, their suitability for the local climate, traffic mix, cost and availability (Box 3.6). In the WHO African Region, more than one third of countries (37%) specify a standard for helmets *(36)*. Helmets for tropical use have been designed for south Asian

Box 3.5 Non-standard motorcycle helmet use in low-and middle-income countries

USE OF NON-STANDARD HELMETS can reduce the effectiveness of helmet-wearing; however, the extent to which such helmets are used has not been assessed. Collaborating institutions in low-and middle-income countries undertook cross-sectional surveys to assess such use and compare the cost of non-standard and standard helmets in market surveys, and reviewed current legislation and enforcement practices. More than 5500 motorcyclists wearing helmets were observed and interviewed.

More than half (54%) were wearing helmets without markers or stickers indicating that the helmet met a recognized standard. Data from retail outlets showed that standard helmets were two to three times more expensive than non-standard helmets, regardless of the outlet type. Inexpensive helmets (costing less than US$ 10) were more likely to be non-standard.

While seven of the nine participating countries had laws prohibiting use of non-standard helmets, few took a comprehensive approach that included prohibiting the manufacture, sale and importation of such helmets. In addition, there was minimal enforcement of the laws.

A holistic approach is needed for helmet-wearing programmes to be effective, including measures to make standardized helmets more affordable, legislation mandating use of standard helmets, requiring their import and prohibiting the sale of non-standard helmets, and enforcement of the laws.

Source: reference *(41)*.

Box 3.6 Selected helmet standards and markings

COUNTRIES THAT HAVE ADOPTED SPECIFIC HELMET STANDARDS have also adopted markings as a way to help consumers purchasing helmets to identify those that meet the required standard. The markings must be difficult to modify in order to prevent counterfeiting.

UNECE Regulation No 22, Uniform provisions concerning the approval of protective helmets and their visors for drivers and passengers of motor cycles and mopeds (E/ECE324-E/ECE/TRANS/505/Rev.1/Add.21)

Australian Standard AS 1698

British Standard BS 6658

Japan Industrial Standard T8133

USA Federal Motor Vehicle Safety StandardNo 218, Motorcycle helmets

and South-East Asian countries with very hot climates. Thailand is considering helmet standards for children *(3)*. Countries that permit children to ride on motorcycles should not only provide an age restriction in their laws but also specify helmet standards for children.

Enforcement and other regulatory measures

Laws and regulations should include enforcement clauses to ensure that they are effective. Lack of clear penalties or enforcement mechanisms can be a barrier. In Viet Nam, regulations governing fines and penalties made it impossible to enforce the helmet-wearing law for children (Box 3.7). Other issues, such as minimum passenger age, add complexity to the enforcement of a helmet-wearing law, by requiring verification of a child's age.

A checklist for assessing the comprehensiveness of motorcycle helmets is contained in Table 3.3.

Box 3.7 Challenges to enforcing child helmet-wearing laws in Viet Nam

RESOLUTION 32 ENACTED IN 2007 mandated the wearing of a helmet by all motorcycle drivers and passengers, with no exemption for children. The law was, however, inconsistent with a higher piece of legislation, the Ordinance for Administrative Sanctions, which made it impossible to enforce helmet-wearing by children, as it prohibits sanctioning of children aged under 14 years. Furthermore, neither piece of legislation provided a mechanism for penalizing adults when a child under their care did not wear a helmet. Children aged 16–18 years could be penalized directly but at half the adult rate while the new law allowed heavy fines–10 times greater than those in previous laws–to be imposed for transporting a child on a motorcycle without a helmet.

The effect of the failure to enforce the legislation for children could be seen in roadside surveys, which revealed that whereas 97% of adults wore helmets 1 year after implementation of Resolution 32, helmet-wearing rates among children were as low as 39%. A legislative working group was formed, with representatives from various government agencies, to draft legislation allowing penalties to be applied to any parent or adult carrying a child on a motorcycle without a helmet.

Sources: references *(42-43)*.

Table 3.3 Checklist for assessing the comprehensiveness of legislation on motorcycle helmets

Does the content of current legislation address:

	Yes	No
1 Helmet use		
Includes compulsory helmet-wearing for all riders (i.e. drivers and passengers)		
Defines helmet-wearing as including proper strapping and wearing of a helmet that meets national standards		
Requires all riders to wear a helmet on all roads		
Requires riders of all motorized two- or three-wheeled motorized vehicles (all engine types) to wear a helmet		
Sets a minimum age for riding a motorcycle		
2 Helmet standards		
Specifies recognized helmet safety standards based on internationally recognized standards		
Includes product labelling requirements and addresses tampering		
Specifies requirements for child helmets (e.g. age or height) depending on the age at which children are allowed to ride on motorcycles		
3 Enforcement		
Specifies who has authority for enforcement		
Allows primary enforcement: no other traffic offence is required to stop a violator and enforce helmet-wearing law		
4 Penalties		
Specifies financial penalties		
Includes provisions for motorcycle impoundment		
5 Other regulatory measures for helmet-wearing		
Establishes penalties for sale of de-specified helmets		
Establishes penalties for tampering with product labelling		
Sets requirements for passenger helmet-wearing for public service two-and three-wheeled motorized vehicles		

3.1.4 Seat-belts

Problem statement

Non-use of seat-belts can result in serious injuries and fatalities. While they do not prevent crashes, seat-belts can reduce the severity of injuries and the number of fatalities by preventing collision with the front seat or steering wheel, preventing complete ejection from the vehicle and distributing the force of the crash over the strongest part of the body *(6)*.

When lap and shoulder belts are used correctly, they reduce the risk of fatal injury among front-seat passengers by 40–50% *(1)*. About 60% of passengers killed in traffic crashes were not wearing their seat-belts, according to the National Highway Traffic Safety Administration (44). While the back seat is the safest place to ride in a car, unbelted back-seat passengers risk serious injury and pose a potentially fatal threat to others during a crash. All passengers, regardless of their seating position, should be properly restrained in a moving vehicle.

Global status of seat-belt legislation

The use of seat-belts has been shown to save lives see (Box 3.8). While many countries have seat-belt laws, they often fail to protect passengers and rear-seat occupants *(1)*. The number of countries with laws that prohibit tampering with seat-belts or that regulate vehicle imports and upgrading requirements is unknown. In Malaysia, where the mandatory rear seat-belt law came into effect on 1 January 2009, the owners of cars registered after 1995 without the belt mountings were given a 3-year grace period to retrofit rear seat-belts *(45)*.

Resources for evidence-based laws and regulations

The UNECE recommends that wearing seat-belts should be required in all motor vehicles in all seating positions (forward- and rear-facing) in which seat-belts are installed. Further, it recommends that seat-belts be fitted at all seating positions in all motor vehicles equipped with anchorage points, in accordance with the latest technical standards. The UNECE also recommends restraints in passenger vehicles with fewer than eight seats, in addition to the driver, such as ISOFIX systems for both seat-belts and child seats *(2)*.

Enforcement and other regulatory measures

Other regulatory measures which could be covered by seat-belt laws include the following:

- *Primary enforcement laws:* These laws allow police officers to stop a vehicle solely for observed violation of the seat-belt law, with no other reason. Secondary enforcement laws allow police to stop a vehicle only if the driver has committed a traffic violation other than not wearing a seat-belt; checking compliance with seat-belt wearing is secondary. Primary enforcement laws are more effective than secondary laws in decreasing fatalities *(46)*, and the rate of seat-belt wearing increases when the law is upgraded from secondary to primary *(47–49)*.

- *Penalties:* Penalties for not wearing a seat-belt should be appropriate and adequate for the country, like other traffic laws, in order to deter noncompliance with the law.

- *Vehicle inspection requirements and vehicle importation laws:* In addition to manufacturing requirements, other regulatory mechanisms must be in place to ensure that vehicles are equipped with seat-belts in working condition. UNECE recommends that seat-belts be inspected as part of vehicle inspections *(2)* and therefore integrated into vehicle inspection regulations. Measures must also be in place to mandate vehicle inspections, with consequences to drivers and owners who avoid or fail inspection and an obligation to remediate defects after inspection.

- *Safe vehicle manufacture:* The Global New Car Assessment Programme (50) provides a platform for sharing best practice among similar programmes around the world and encouraging the manufacture of safer motor vehicles globally. This Programme and other regional programmes such as the New Car Assessment Programme in the Latin American and Caribbean region (Latin NCAP) *(51)* can help consumers by developing crash test programmes in emerging markets where vehicle growth is strong but independent consumer information is frequently not available.

Box 3.8 Seat-belts save lives

A COMPREHENSIVE SEAT-BELT LAW would include provisions mandating the fitting and wearing of seat-belts of a given standard in all vehicles. In 1961, the State of Wisconsin in the USA introduced a law requiring seat-belts to be fitted in the front of vehicles. Victoria and South Australia followed suit in 1964, as did the rest of Australia in subsequent years. Europe made seat-belts mandatory in 1965. While much of the world has followed these good practices, a significant number of countries have yet to do so. According to the 2013 *Global Status report on road safety*, only 111 countries reported having seat-belt laws covering all occupants.

Mandatory seat-belt laws, when enforced, save lives. According to the US National Highway Traffic Safety Administration in seat-belts save the lives of 10 000 people each year. In 2009, over 33 000 people were killed and 2.2 million injured in motor vehicle crashes. More than 70% were in the passenger seats of vehicles and trucks, and more than half were not restrained at the time of the crash. Mandatory seat-belt laws, education and technology for restraint systems increased seat-belt use in the USA from 11% in 1981 to nearly 85% in 2010, saving hundreds of thousands of lives. While there is increasing use of seat-belts in the USA, one in seven people still do not 'buckle up', indicating that more needs to be done.

Sources: references *(1, 45)*.

Lives saved by seat-belt usage in the USA

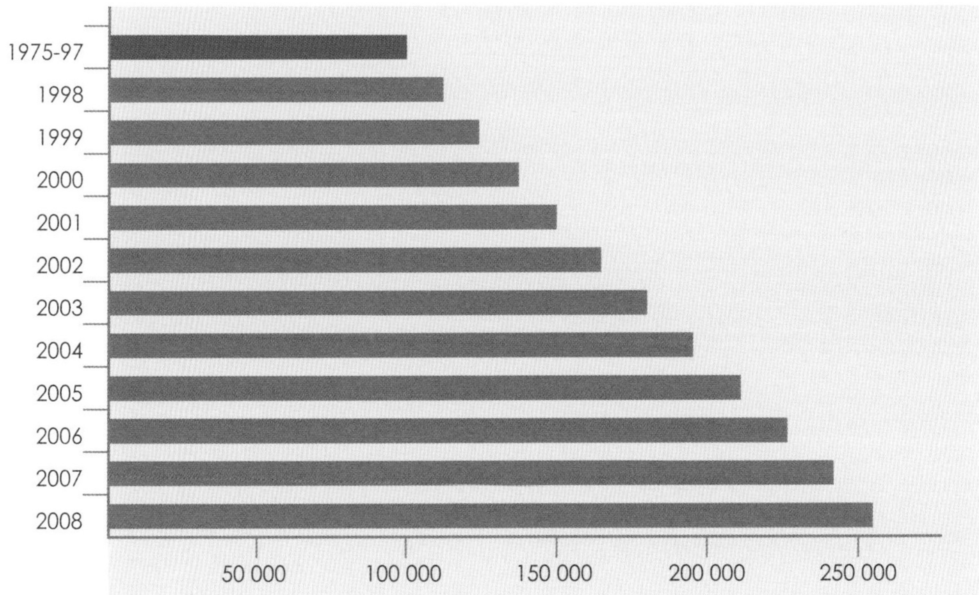

Cumulative number of lives saved by seat-belts in the USA

UNECE recommendations for periodic inspection of vehicles include checks on safety belts and buckles. The security of the mounting should be inspected visually and rejected if the anchorage point is badly deteriorated. The condition of a seat-belt should be checked both visually and by operating it. The vehicle should be rejected if mandatory seat-belts are missing or not fitted, if the belt is damaged or not in accordance with the regulations and if the buckle or the retractor is damaged or not functioning correctly *(2)*. A checklist for assessing the comprehensiveness of seat-belt legislation in contained in Table 3.4.

Table 3.4 Checklist for assessing the comprehensiveness of seat-belt legislation

Does the content of current legislation address:

	Yes	No
1 Mandatory seat-belt laws for all occupants		
2 Manufacturing standards		
Includes seat–belt requirements		
Sets standards for imported vehicles		
Prohibits de-specification		
Sets retro-fitting requirements for older vehicles and phase-in period		
3 Enforcement		
Specifies who has authority for enforcement		
Specifies primary versus secondary enforcement		
4 Penalties		
Specifies financial penalties for not wearing a seat-belt		
5 Other regulatory measures for seat belts		
Prohibits carrying more passengers than seating positions and overloading		
Requires periodic inspection		

3.1.5 Child restraints

Problem statement

It has been shown that properly restraining children in vehicles reduces injuries and fatalities in the event of a crash (Box 3.9); yet many children are transported without restraints. Child restraints are expensive and inaccessible in many low-income countries, where the number of injuries and fatalities is in general higher. One practical reason for noncompliance is lack of space for a child safety seat, especially in vehicles that transport large families or crowded public service vehicles. A law requiring child restraints might therefore be aspirational in some countries.

Global status of child restraint legislation

According to the 2013 *Global status report on road safety (1)*, 88% of high-income countries and only 30% of low-income countries have national laws on child restraints. Even in countries with laws, however, restraints are often of the wrong type or are inappropriately used, or the law is inadequately enforced. Child restraints are incorrectly used in 15–80% of cases, because either the belt is not properly fastened, the child seat is incorrectly installed or the belt is placed around a child's neck, under the arms or across the abdomen *(52)*.

Resources for evidence-based laws and regulations

Both the UNECE *(2)* and WHO *(1)* recommend that countries enact legislation requiring that children be properly secured in a restraint system and seated in the proper position (forward- or rear-facing) when being transported in a vehicle and that the restraint should take into account the child's age, height and weight. The UNECE also recommends that countries require the use of only approved child restraint systems and consider prohibiting sale of restraints that do not meet the standard for use in vehicles. Examples of child restraint requirements are listed in Table 3.5.

Box 3.9 Saving children's lives by the use of child restraints

MANY STUDIES SHOW THAT CHILD RESTRAINTS reduce fatal injuries among infants by around 70% and by about 54% among children aged 1–4 years. In the USA, the lives of nearly 9000 children were saved by child restraints between 1975 and 2008. Despite the introduction of a law requiring that children be appropriately restrained when travelling in a vehicle, the use of child restraints is by no means universal. For instance, in 2008, child restraints saved an estimated 244 lives. If however, child restraint use had been 100%, 323 lives would have been saved. Thus, the lives of 79 children were lost unnecessarily.

Source: reference *(45)*.

Children's lives saved by child restraint usage in the USA

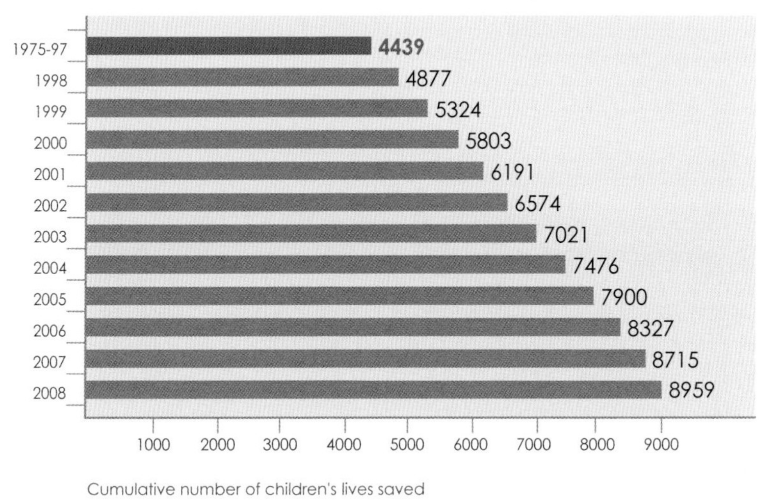

Table 3.5 Child restraint guidelines in Ontario (Canada), South Africa and the USA

Ontario, South Africa and the USA have classified child restraint systems by law into three categories: rear-facing infant restraints, child restraints and booster seats.

Canada (Ontario)	South Africa	USA
Birth to 9 kg Rear-facing seat away from an active airbag.	**Birth to12 months** Keep child in rear-facing seat, until the child is at least 12 months old and weighs at least 9 kg.	**Birth to12 months** Car seats for infants must be rear-facing; the height and weight limits for the rear-facing position in convertible and three-in-one seats are usually higher, so that a child can be kept in the rear-facing position for longer.
Children weighing 9–18 kg: Forward-facing seat with a tether strap.	**Children 1–4 years** Children ≥ 1 year weighing 9–18 kg who can no longer ride in rear-facing seats should ride in forward-facing child safety seats until either their weight exceeds 18 kg or they grow too tall for the height of the adjustable harness.	**Children 1–3 years** Children should remain in rear-facing car seats until they reach the height or weight limit allowed by the car seat manufacturer. They can then travel in a forward-facing car seat with a harness.
Pre-school to 8 years Booster seats are required for children < 8 years weighing ≥ 18 kg but < 36 kg and are < 145 cm tall.	**Children 4–6 years** Booster seats are used only when a child has outgrown a safety seat designed for those weighing 15–25 kg. Children should ride in a booster seat until the lap and diagonal belts of car seats fit properly, usually when they are about 145 cm tall. Booster cushions without backs are designed for children weighing 22–36 kg; manufacturers now produce booster cushions with backs suitable for children weighing 15–36 kg. Shield booster seats, which have a plastic shield in front of the child, offer less protection and should not be used. Children weighing > 18 kg should be correctly secured in belt-positioning boosters or other appropriate restraints until adult lap and shoulder belts fit correctly, usually around age 8 years.	**Children 3–7 years** A child should be kept in a forward-facing car seat with a harness until he or she reaches the height or weight limit allowed by the manufacturer. Once children outgrow forward-facing car seats with a harness, they can travel in a booster seat, but still in the back seat.
Youth Children can start using a seat belt once they weigh 36 kg, measure 145 cm or are 8 years old. Each child should wear a seat belt.	**Children 8 years and over** Once a child's eyes are level with the top of the back seat of the car or the child weighs ≥ 26 kg, he or she may use a seat belt. The seat belt must fit the child correctly, with the lap belt low over the bony part of the hips (not the stomach) and the sash not touching the face or neck when all slack is removed. Indicators of a good fit.	**Children 8–12 years** Children should be kept in a booster seat until they are large enough to fit in a seat belt properly. For a seat belt to fit properly, the lap belt must lie snugly across the upper thighs, not the stomach. The shoulder belt must lie snugly across the shoulder and chest and not cross the neck or face. Children should still ride in the back seat.

Source: adapted from references *(53-55)*.

Choosing a proper car seat is important. As there are many child restraints on the market, regulations should specify use of an approved child restraint, which is specifically manufactured for children and meets safety standards.

Enforcement and other regulatory measures

UNECE Regulation 44 *(56)* provides technical requirements for child restraint systems suitable for use in power-driven vehicles with three or more wheels, based on the child's seating position, age, height and weight, according to the following five categories:

- group 0 for children of a mass less than 10 kg;
- group 0+ for children of a mass less than 13 kg;
- group I for children of mass from 9 kg to 18 kg;
- group II for children of mass from 15 kg to 25 kg;
- group III for children of mass from 22 kg to 36 kg.

A checklist for assessing the comprehensiveness of child restraint legislation is contained in Table 3.6.

Table 3.6 Checklist for assessing the comprehensiveness of child restraint legislation

Does the content of current legislation address:

	Yes	No
1 Use of child restraints		
Mandatory use of child restraints appropriate for age, height and weight		
Positioning: forward- versus rear-facing		
Carriage of children in front seats		
Child restraint standards and product labelling		
2 Enforcement		
Primary versus secondary enforcement		
3 Penalties		
Financial penalties		
Other penalties		
4 Other regulatory mechanisms		
Any other measures		

Chapter 3 Practice and resources

3.2 Improving the comprehensiveness of laws relevant to post-crash care

According to European studies, about 50% of all road traffic deaths occur within a few minutes either at the crash scene or on the way to the hospital *(57)*. Prompt, good quality pre-hospital care can save the lives of many injured persons *(1)*, and deaths that result from road crashes could be prevented with improved response *(58, 59)*. Access to the essential elements for preventing deaths and improving recovery varies greatly, because of weak public health infrastructure, especially in low- and middle-income countries. The elements include lack of help at the crash scene and proper care before arriving at the hospital, lack of access to emergency medical services, lack of personnel trained in trauma care and lack of rehabilitation and psychosocial care *(57)*.

As post-crash care is only one component of an overall trauma care system, studies should be conducted to determine how the emergency or trauma care system looks after injured people in general, how crash events fit into the overall system and whether laws and regulations are in place to support care of the injured. A country's trauma care system is also part of broader emergency and disaster preparedness. The recommended steps to be taken are:

- Step 1: Conduct a rapid assessment of the trauma care system and existing laws.
- Step 2: Determine gaps in post-crash care laws and how to improve them.

3.2.1 Conduct a rapid assessment of the trauma care system

Post-crash care can be classified into three main categories: pre-hospital care, hospital care and rehabilitation. Its main goals are to avoid death, to limit the severity of injuries, to avoid sequelae such as long-term disability and to ensure the best possible recovery and reintegration into society *(15)*. A situational assessment can identify gaps in laws governing these three health-care categories and also ways in which they can be strengthened by comparing them with laws in countries with mature trauma care systems.

The 'trauma system maturity index' (Table 3.7) is a simple tool for conducting a rapid assessment of the trauma system in a district, province or country. It can indicate the action required by managers and planners to improve the system, and allows broad comparisons of trauma systems. Trauma systems are graded from level I (least mature) to level IV (most mature).

The trauma system maturity index can serve as the basis for determining the legislative and regulatory framework required to improve post-crash care (see Table 3.8).

3.2.2 Ensure a comprehensive regulatory and legislative framework for post-crash care

When deciding on the laws required for comprehensive post-crash care, it is useful to examine the laws in place in other countries at a similar level of maturity with regard to trauma care in order to identify any gaps. It can also be useful to examine the laws in countries with mature post-crash care systems to identify goals. Examination of laws within a region can help in normalization.

Laws on emergency medical services in countries in Europe differ with respect to how long they have been in place and what they address. About one third were issued in the 1990s and more than half in the 2000s. The topics addressed include free access to hospital care, including for uninsured and unidentified people; minimum standards of care and equipment; minimum qualification requirements; financing mechanisms; and required training for operating staff *(60)*.

Both in the European Union and elsewhere, laws are not always set by national legislation but may consist of regulations drawn up by legislatively created entities with the responsibility to regulate various aspects of trauma care, such as professional licensing and accrediting bodies. In 2007 in India, for example, the Gujarat Assembly adopted an emergency medical services law that established state authority for such services and instructed city and district councils to prepare plans for and ensure provision of services. Their responsibilities include contracting hospitals that meet minimum staffing requirements; establishing ambulance requirements, including equipment, supplies and staff; and setting penalties for violation of the law *(61)*. Under South Africa's Health Professions Act, no person, educational institution or training facility can offer education and training for the purposes of qualifying a person in the practice of any health profession, unless the education and training has been accredited by the appropriate professional board, such as the Professional Board for Emergency Care *(62)*.

As for all aspects of road safety, strengthening the regulatory framework for emergency services and post-crash requires collaboration among various government agencies. In Romania's Health System Reform Law of 2006, emergency care is defined as a duty of the state, and the law authorizes the Ministry of Health to further regulate the area of trauma

Table 3.7 Trauma system maturity index

	Level I	Level II	Level III	Level IV
Pre-hospital trauma care	No mapping of pre-hospital resources, no formal emergency medical services, lack of availability or duplication of pre-hospital services, no defined communication system.	Pre-hospital resources identifiable, no coordination between public and private providers of pre-hospital care, no universal access number, weak communication.	Formal emergency medical services, universal access number available, coordination among various agencies for pre-hospital care, well defined communication.	Formal emergency medical services controlled by a lead agency, national universal access number, legislative mechanism in place to govern emergency medical services and allow universal coverage.
Education and training	No identified health personnel to offer primary trauma care in the community.	Identified health personnel in the community for emergency trauma care, no definite training requirements for health workers or ambulance personnel.	Health professionals and paramedics trained in providing emergency trauma care, trauma training courses available.	Educational standards and training for emergency trauma care providers laid down, licensing and renewal norms for different levels of paramedics in place.
Facility trauma care	Role of secondary and tertiary facilities unclear, health facilities lack human and physical resources, no clear referral linkages.	Roles of various health care facilities clear, referral linkages present, no documentation or needs assessment of facilities as per *Guidelines for essential trauma care*[a], no lead agency in the system.	Health facilities in the systems are assessed as per *Guidelines for essential trauma care*[a], and documented human and physical resources are available and ensured around the clock, lead agency present.	Mechanism for hospital verification and accreditation in place through ministry of health or professional bodies, lead agency with mandate to supervise trauma care.
Quality assurance	No injury surveillance or registry mechanism in place to obtain comprehensive data.	Injury data available, but no formal attempt to document or analyse them, no initiative for quality assurance.	Basic quality assurance programme as per *Guidelines for essential trauma care*[a] in place.	Formal quality assurance programme in place and mandated in pre-hospital and facility services.

[a] Mock C et al. Guidelines for essential trauma care. Geneva, World Health Organization, 2004.

Source: reference (63).

care. The Ministry of Health, with input from a consultative committee, drafted regulations covering staffing levels, physical resources and financing. In partnership with the Ministry of Interior, which oversees fire departments, the Ministry of Health issued interministerial decree 1092/1500/2006, which set criteria for several types of ambulance vehicles, from first-response vehicles to mobile intensive care units, and for the competence of ambulance personnel. Logistic and safety regulations were created and a partnership established with the police force for enforcing the standards through spot checks *(64)*.

Table 3.8 lists topics that have been covered in laws and regulations on post-crash care in various countries, including victims' compensation, insurance and data collection and reporting. Recommendations from international organizations are also included.

Examples of various laws and regulations covering such issues from a range of countries are provided for reference in the attached Annex.

Table 3.8 Areas of a trauma care system that could be addressed in legislation

Topic	Regulatory topics that could be addressed
Pre-hospital trauma care	Duty to assist the injured (see Annex A.5.a)
	Protection of individuals who assist the injured, i.e. so-called 'good samaritan' laws (see Annex A.5.b)
	Ambulance and emergency vehicle requirements (see Annex A.5.c)
	First-aid training as a prerequisite for licensure for driving certain classes of vehicle (see Annex A.5.d)
	Requirements for contents of first-aid kits (see Annex A.5.d)
Education and training	Creation or designation of an entity responsible for regulating educational and licensure requirements for direct care providers and scope of practice requirements
Facility trauma care	Duty to provide treatment and stabilization and to transfer a patient (see Annex A.5.e)
	Mandating emergency department accreditation requirements and creation or designation of an entity responsible for accreditation
Quality assurance	Creation or designation of an independent entity responsible for monitoring the quality of pre-hospital and rehabilitation services
	Data reporting requirements to ensure proper monitoring and feedback on quality of services
Other	Victims' compensation (see Annex A.5.f)
	Third-party insurance requirements
	Maintenance of records, disclosure and other confidentiality requirements

Source: adapted from reference *(63)*.

3.3 References

1. *Global status report on road safety:* supporting a decade of action. Geneva, World health Organization, 2013.

2. *Consolidated Resolution on Road Traffic, 14 August 2009.* Geneva, United Nations Economic Commission for Europe, Working Party on Road Traffic Safety, 2010 (ECE/TRANS/WP.1/123).

3. *Helmets: a roadsafety manual for decision-makers and practitioners.* Geneva, World Health Organization, 2006.

4. *Drinking and driving: a road safety manual for decision-makers and practitioners.* Geneva, Global Road Safety Partnership, 2007.

5. *Speed management: a road safety manual for decision-makers and practitioners.* Geneva, Global Road Safety Partnership, 2008.

6. *Seat-belts and child restraints: a road safety-manual for decision-makers and practitioners.* London, FIA Foundation for the Automobile and Society 2009.

7. *Data systems: a road safety manual for decision-makers and practitioners.* Geneva, World Health Organization, 2010.

8. Tefft B. Impact speed and a pedestrian's risk of severe injury or death. *Accident Analysis and Prevention,* 2013, 50: 871–878.

9. Davis GA. Relating severity of pedestrian injury to impact speed in vehicle pedestrian crashes. *Transportation Research Record,* 2001, 1773: 108–113.

10. Rosén E, Stigson H, Sander U. Literature review of pedestrian fatality risk as a function of car impact speed. *Accident Analysis and Prevention,* 2011, 43: 25–33.

11. *Towards zero: ambitious road safety targets and the safe systems approach.* Paris, Organisation for Economic Co-operation and Development, International Transport Forum 2008.

12. Wilson C et al. Speed cameras for the prevention of road traffic injuries and deaths. *Cochrane Database of Systematic Reviews,* 2011, Issue 2.

13. Hickman JS et al. *Safety impacts of speed limiter device installations on commercial trucks and buses.* Washington DC, The National Academies Press, 2009 (Commercial Truck and Bus Safety Synthesis Program Report No. 16).

14. Allsopp R. *The effectiveness of speed cameras. A review of the literature.* London, RAC Foundation, 2010 (http://www.racfoundation.org/research/safety/effectiveness-of-speed-cameras, accessed 10 January 2013).

15. Peden M et al., eds. *World report on road traffic injury prevention.* Geneva, World Health Organization, 2004.

16. Allsop RE. *Alcohol and road accidents: a discussion of the Grand Rapids study.* Harmondsworth, Road Research Laboratory, 1966 (RRL Report No. 6).

17. Borkenstein RF et al. *The role of the drinking driver in traffic accidents.* Bloomington, IN, Department of Police Administration, Indiana University, 1964.

18. Moskowitz H et al. Methodological issues in epidemiological studies of alcohol crash risk. In: Mayhew DR, Dussault C, eds. *Proceedings of the 16th International Conference on Alcohol, Drugs and Traffic Safety, Montreal, 4–9 August 2002.* Montreal, Société de l'Assurance Automobile du Québec, 2002:45–50 (http://www.saaq.gouv.qc.ca/t2002/actes/pdf/(06a).pdf, accessed 10 January 2013).

19. Compton RP et al. Crash risk of alcohol impaired driving. In: Mayhew DR, Dussault C, eds. *Proceedings of the 16th International Conference on Alcohol, Drugs and Traffic Safety, Montreal, 4–9 August 2002.* Montreal, Société de l'Assurance Automobile du Québec, 2002:39–44 (http://www.saaq.gouv.qc.ca/t2002/actes/pdf/(06a).pdf, accessed 10 January 2013).

20. Zwerling C, Jones P. Evaluation of the effectiveness of low blood alcohol concentration laws for younger drivers. *American Journal of Preventive Medicine,* 1999, 16:76–80.

21. Senserrick T. Australian graduated driver licensing systems. *Journal of the Australasian College of Road Safety*, 2009, 20:20–26.

22. Magnusson P, Jakobsson L, Hultman S. Alcohol interlock systems in Sweden: 10 years of systematic work. *American Journal of Preventive Medicine*, 2011; 40:378–379.

23. Babor T et al. *Alcohol: no ordinary commodity.* New York, Oxford University Press, 2010:166–183.

24. Peek-Asa C. The effect of random alcohol screening in reducing motor vehicle crash injuries. *American Journal of Preventive Medicine*, 1999, 16 (1S):57–67.

25. Shults RA et al. Reviews of evidence regarding interventions to reduce alcohol-impaired driving. *American Journal of Preventive Medicine*, 2001, 21:66–88.

26. Hingson RW et al. Interventions to prevent alcohol-related injuries. In Doll LS et al., eds. *Handbook of injury and violence prevention.* New York, Springer, 2007:295–310.

27. *Global status report on alcohol and health.* Geneva, World Health Organization, 2011 (http://www.who.int/substance_abuse/publications/global_alcohol_report/en/, accessed 10 January 2013).

28. Government of South Africa. *The National Road Traffic Act, 1996 (Act No. 93 of 1996) [Actsonline web site].* (http://www.acts.co.za/rt_nrta/index.htm, accessed 10 January 2013).

29. *The Criminal Law (Forensic Procedures) Amendment Act*, 2010, Section 37. Cape Town, Government of South Africa 2010 (http://www.justice.gov.za/legislation/acts/acts_full.html, accessed 10 January 2013).

30. Motor Vehicles Act 1988. New Delhi, Ministry of Road Transport and Highways, 1988 (http://www.morth.nic.in/index2.asp?slid=95&sublinkid=54&lang=1, accessed 9 January 2013).

31. *South Australia Road Traffic Act of 1961*, Section 47. Adelaide, Government of South Australia, 1961 (http://www.legislation.sa.gov.au/lz/c/a/road%20traffic%20act%201961.aspx, accessed 10 January 2013).

32. Willis C, Lybrand S, Bellamy M. Alcohol ignition interlock programmes for reducing drink driving recidivism. *Cochrane Database of Systematic Reviews*, 2009, Issue 1.

33. Elder RW et al. Effectiveness of ignition interlocks for preventing alcohol-impaired driving and alcohol-related crashes. A community guide systematic review. *American Journal of Preventive Medicine*, 2011, 40:362–376.

34. Bjerre B. Primary and secondary prevention of drink driving by the use of Alcolock device and program: Swedish experiences. *Accident Analysis and Prevention*, 2005, 37:1145–1152.

35. Lahausse JA, Fieldes BN. Cost–benefit analysis of an alcohol ignition interlock for installation in all newly registered vehicles. *Traffic Injury Prevention*, 2009, 10:528–537.

36. *Status report on road safety in countries of the WHO African Region.* Brazzaville, World Health Organization Regional Office for Africa, 2010 (http://www.afro.who.int/en/clusters-a-programmes/dpc/mental-health-violence-and-injuries/features/2846-status-report-on-road-safety-in-countries-of-the-who-african-region.html, accessed 10 January 2013).

37. Kumar A, Barrett F. *Africa Infrastructure Country Diagnostic. Stuck in traffic: urban transport in Africa. Summary of background paper 1.* World Bank and the Sub-Saharan Africa Transport Policy Program, The World Bank, 2008 (http://www.eu-africa-infrastructure-tf.net/attachments/library/aicd-background-paper-1-urban-trans-summary-en.pdf, accessed 10 January 2013).

38. Kumar A. *Understanding the emerging role of motorcycles in African cities. A political economy perspective. Sub-Saharan African Transport Policy Program (SSATP) Discussion Paper No. 13.* (Urban Transport Series). World Bank and SSATP, 2011 (http://siteresources.worldbank.org/EXTAFRSUBSAHTRA/Resources/1513929-1262811948762/DP13-Role-Motorcycles.pdf, accessed 10 January 2013).

39. Liu B et al. Helmets for preventing injury in motorcycle riders. *Cochrane Database of Systematic Reviews*, 2009, Issue 1.

40. *Regulation No. 22-Rev. 4-Protective helmets and their visors for drivers and passengers of motor cycles and mopeds.* Geneva, United Nations Economic Commission for Europe, 2002 (http://www.unece.org/trans/main/wp29/wp29regs21-40.html, accessed 10 January 2013).

41. Road Traffic Injury Research Network Multicentre Study Collaborators et al. The use of non-standard motorcycle helmets in low- and middle-income countries: a multicentre study. *Injury Prevention,* 2012, 0:1-6.

42. Passmore J et al. The formulation and implementation of a national helmet law: a case study for Viet Nam. *Bulletin of the World Health Organization*, 2010, 88:783–787.

43. Pervin A et al. Viet Nam's mandatory motorcycle helmet law and its impact on children. *Bulletin of the World Health Organization*, 2009, 87:369–373.

44. *Policy impact.* Seat-belts. Atlanta, GA, Centers for Disease Control and Prevention National Center for Injury Prevention and Control, Division of Unintentional Injury Prevention (http://www.cdc.gov/MotorVehicleSafety/pdf/PolicyImpact-SeatBelts.pdf, accessed 10 January 2013).

45. *Research Report. Phase 1: Achievements of First 3-Month Advocacy Program. Rear Seatbelt Use: Public Awareness and Practice*. Kajang, Malaysian Institute of Road Safety Research (MIROS), 2008 (http://miros.gov.my/web/guest/reports, accessed 11 January 2013).

46. Dellinger A et al. Interventions to prevent motor vehicle injuries. In: Doll LS et al., eds. *Handbook of injury and violence prevention*, New York, Springer, 2007:55–79.

47. Farmer CM, Williams AF. Effect on fatality risk of changing from secondary to primary seat-belt enforcement. *Journal of Safety Research*, 2005, 36:189–194.

48. Shults RA et al. Primary enforcement seat-belt laws are effective even in the face of rising belt use rates. *Accident Analysis and Prevention*, 2004, 36(3):491–493.

49. Dinh-Zarr TB et al. Reviews of evidence regarding interventions to increase the use of safety belts. *American Journal of Preventive Medicine*, 2001, 21:48–65.

50. Global New Car Assessment Programme [web site home page] (http://www.globalncap.org/Pages/HomeMain.aspx, accessed 10 January 2013).

51. Latin American and Caribbean New Car Assessment Programme [web site home page] (http://www.latinncap.com/en/about-us, accessed 10 January 2013).

52. Elvik R et al. *The handbook of road safety measures*. New York, Emerald Publishing, 2009:609–615.

53. *Safe & secure: choosing the right car seat for your child.* Toronto, Ontario Ministry of Transportation (http://www.mto.gov.on.ca/english/safety/carseat/choose.shtml, accessed 10 January 2013).

54. *Car seat recommendations for children.* Washington, DC, National Highway Safety Traffic Administration (http://www.nhtsa.gov/Safety/CPS, accessed 10 January 2013).

55. *Arrive alive*. Pretoria, Government of South Africa [web site home page] (http://www.arrivealive.co.za/pages.aspx?i=1523, accessed 10 January 2013).

56. *Regulation No. 44. –Revision 2. Uniform Provisions Concerning the Approval of Restraining Devices for Child Occupants of Power-Driven Vehicles ("Child Restraint System")*,Geneva.United Nations Economic Commission for Europe, (http://www.unece.org/trans/main/wp29/wp29regs41-60.html, accessed 9 January 2013).

57. Buylaert W, ed. *Reducing injuries from post-impact care.* Brussels, European Transport Safety Council Working Party on Post Impact Care, 1999.

58. Mock CN, nii-Amon-Kotei D, Maier RV. Low utilization of formal medical services by injured persons in a developing nation: health service data underestimate the importance of trauma. *Journal of Trauma*, 1997, 42:504–513.

59. Hussain IM, Redmond AD. Are pre-hospital deaths from accidental injury preventable? *British Medical Journal*, 1994, 308:1077–1080.

60. *Emergency medical services systems in the European Union*. Geneva, World Health Organization, World Health Organization, 2008

61. *Gujarat Emergency Medical Services Act of 2007. Government of Gujarat, Health and Family Welfare Department*, (http://www.gujhealth.gov.in/related-act-rules.htm, accessed 10 January 2013).

62. *Health Professions Act of 1974*. Pretoria, Government of South Africa (http://www.acts.co.za/health_professions_act_1974/index.htm, accessed 10 January 2013).

63. *Trauma system maturity index*. Geneva, World Health Organization, [web site home page] (http://www.who.int/violence_injury_prevention/services/traumacare/maturity_index/en/index.html, accessed 10 January 2013).

64. *Strengthening care for the injured: success stories and lessons learned from around the world*. Geneva, World Health Organization, 2010 (http://whqlibdoc.who.int/publications/2010/9789241563963_eng.pdf, accessed 10 January 2013).

Chapter 4

Advocating for legislative and regulatory change

Chapter 4 Advocating for legislative and regulatory change

Advocacy can be defined as 'a set of targeted actions directed at decision-makers in support of a specific policy issue' *(1)*. It is important to plan advocacy properly in order to bring about legislative change; the recommended steps for planning an advocacy campaign are as follows:

- Identify the issue to be addressed.
- Set advocacy goals and objectives.
- Know the political landscape.
- Design and convey effective messages.
- Cultivate policy champions, and build strong partnerships.
- Create an action plan, implement, and monitor progress *(1)*.

Although these steps need not be completed in the order presented, all are essential.

4.1 Identify the issue to be addressed

The first step in advocacy is to identify the problem or issue and its context. Issues may arise from a rising incidence or prevalence of road crashes and concomitant injuries and fatalities, which may in turn precipitate public outcry, a demand for change, government-initiated road safety law reform, national commitment to a global action plan or implementation of a national road safety plan.

Not all road safety issues require legislative change. Some simply require implementation or enforcement of existing laws by changing societal norms and values or by strengthening capacity or resources. In this manual, the road safety issues are limited to those that require legislation or regulation.

In addition, priorities must be set. There may be many problems, but the resources to address them may be limited and must be taken into account in setting priorities. The list of priorities should also take into account the importance, urgency, magnitude and impact of each problem nationally.

4.2 Set advocacy goals and objectives

Setting clear goals and objectives is an indispensable part of advocacy. Ultimately, the goal should be comprehensive laws, which, together with social marketing to change behaviour and consistent, sustained enforcement, will reduce road traffic-related injuries and fatalities. Other, similar goals can be set. Often, the goal is for greater road safety in general, legislative improvements being but one means of achieving this aim. The objectives should be measurable, so that their progress can be evaluated. For example, the objectives of helmet legislation might be:

- to amend the law to mandate the wearing of approved standard helmets within 2 years;
- within 2 years, to propose a new law making the wearing of helmets that meet an approved standard compulsory for all riders and passengers of motorcycles of all engines, on all road types.

4.3 Know the political landscape

Knowing the political landscape means understanding the legislative and regulatory process and who the key players are. Political ideologies and systems significantly influence the success of legislative change. Understanding the governance system helps to define the approach to take in advocating for legislative change. For example, the levels of participation of the public, private and other sectors in the legislative process determine who should be involved and the point in the process at which their engagement will be most effective. Similarly, a clear understanding of the process of drafting laws and regulations is useful for determining at which stage advocacy will be most effective. Identifying the institutions or individuals that can positively or negatively influence an issue will help in deciding whether to ally with them or be prepared to counter their messages.

Having this information can save time and resources and ensures that advocacy is targeted most effectively. Political mapping involves gathering information about the institutions involved in law-making on road safety, their authority to propose legislation and the procedures for approaching and working with them. Such institutions include parliaments, government bodies, state agencies with power to draft subsidiary legislation or subnational laws (e.g. in federal systems) and counties or municipalities that enact subnational laws or by-laws. Understanding each institution's standing orders and rules of debate will help inform decisions about which advocacy tools to use.

4.3.1 Understand the legislative (or regulatory) process

In general, advocacy should start early, as much of the work on new laws or amendments begins well before a bill reaches parliament or subsidiary legislation is passed by law-making entities. Once a bill enters the formal process, there may still be opportunities to influence its content. The description of Kenya's legislative process given in Box 4.1 illustrates how a pending bill can be influenced at different stages and the opportunities for input from experts and other stakeholders.

Advocacy for legislative change should be targeted, such as:

- a proposal for new legislation or amendment of an existing law to cover a specific risk factor;
- to repeal or comprehensively overhaul an existing road safety law or regulation;
- a proposal for subsidiary (secondary) legislation by a public agency, such as regulations on use of helmets.

Technical experts in road safety and in legislative drafting can ensure that the content of the proposed changes is comprehensive and is presented in an acceptable form. The WHO document, Advocating for Road Safety and Road Traffic Victims provides guiding principles for advocacy *(2)*.

4.3.2 Map stakeholders

Various government institutions, advocacy organizations and civil society are involved in the processes leading up to legislative or regulatory change. Identifying these entities, their positions on an issue, their strengths and weaknesses and opportunities for forming partnerships allows proper planning of advocacy. In particular, it is helpful to obtain the following information about nongovernmental and other potential stakeholders:

- which organizations are present in the country and the primary contact;
- the type of organization (e.g. a public health association, professional association);
- the organization's focus, (e.g. road safety, transport and mobility, public health, trauma care, engineering);
- the geographical level at which it operates– national, regional or local;
- its main activities and strengths, (e.g. specific road safety interventions, lobbying government for legislative change, conducting public campaigns, events, education and training, research).

Once the stakeholders have been identified, it is important to ascertain their level of influence and role in the legislative process in order to identify the targets of advocacy messages. The questions that can be used to obtain such information include *(1)*:

- Is the individual a key decision-maker?
- What influence does he or she have and at what level?
- What is his or her role in the process, (e.g. vote on issues, make decisions in parliament, on a parliamentary committee, in a government ministry)?
- What is the individual's position on the objective? Is he or she a champion, a potential champion or neutral with respect to the issues and objectives?
- Do you have access to the person, formally or informally, or do you know others who do? Informal access, such as within a community, increases the chances of an encounter and of engaging the individual on a personal level.

Box 4.1 Kenya's legislative process

LEGISLATION IN KENYA entails various processes or stages that present opportunities for intervention by the media and other non-state actors.

Stage 1. Initiation of bills

In Kenya, bills can be initiated by the Government (through ministries) or members of parliament (private Members' Bills) or by petitions from members of the public to the Speaker of the National Assembly.

Stage 2. Publication of bills

Once a bill is drafted, it is published in the *Kenya Gazette*, so that members of the public have an opportunity to scrutinize it. Some bills are published by cabinet secretaries or members of parliament without a commitment to follow the entire process. Published sources of information about bills include:

- the *Kenya Gazette* or the Kenya law reports (available at the web site: www.Kenyalaw.org);
- public officials;
- commentaries from experts in the field;
- the member of parliament proposing the bill;
- non-state actors involved in policy, such as ASIRT-Kenya for Road Safety Laws;
- international and multilateral agencies such as WHO and the United Nations, (for international best practice relevant to the proposed policy).

Stage 3. First reading

A bill is normally tabled before the House and read for the first time. There is no debate on the bill at this stage, which is the first formal step. The bill is then committed to the appropriate departmental committee. For example, the 2012 Traffic Amendment Bill sponsored by the Honourable Jakoyo Midiwo, MP, was committed to the Departmental Committee on Transport, Public Works and Housing. Sources of information about a bill's first reading include:

- the Order Paper, which is the House business agenda for the following day, and can be accessed from Parliament's web site at www.parliament.go.ke;
- the Hansard of the day, which records when the bill was read for the first time;
- the Office of the Clerk of the National Assembly.

Stage 4. Committee stage

During the committee stage, the departmental committee scrutinizes the bill to ensure that it:

- conforms with the Constitution;
- addresses the intended policy issues;
- is not in conflict with other laws.

The departmental committee invites the main stakeholders (public or private) to make presentations on the bill. Any member of the public may request to appear before the committee to make a presentation. This is a critical stage, as the committee then prepares its report on the bill, and makes recommendations on areas for amendment or improvement. Stakeholders should therefore ensure that their proposals form part of the report of the committee. The committee has 10 days to conduct its business and report to the House; however, it usually takes longer to ensure wide stakeholder consultation. It is at this stage that advocacy can be targeted at the appropriate cabinet secretary (or member of parliament if it is a private Member's bill), to support or refute any proposals in the bill. Sources of information during the committee stage include:

- the chairperson of the departmental committee;
- the Office of the Clerk of the National Assembly;
- the relevant cabinet secretary;
- the member of parliament who sponsored the bill.

Continued overleaf

Box 4.1 Kenya's legislative process, continued

Stage 5. Second reading

The bill is then read for the second time. The sponsor and the seconder of the bill are given the opportunity to explain its objectives, and all members of the House can make contributions in support of or opposition to the bill (with or without reservations). At this stage, it is usually possible to guage whether the bill will go through or if it will be rejected. Sources of information for second readings include:

- the Order Paper, which is the House business agenda for the following day available at: (www.parliament.go.ke);
- the Hansard of the day, which summarizes the reading available at: (www.parliament.go.ke);
- the Office of the Clerk of the National Assembly;
- commentaries by experts;
- commentaries by public officials on areas of concern;
- comments by the member of parliament who proposed the bill;
- non-state actors involved in the policy area, such as nongovernmental organizations working on road safety;
- international and multilateral agencies, such as WHO and the United Nations, (for international best practice related to the proposed policy);
- members of the public who are affected by the issues addressed in the bill or are likely to benefit if the law is enacted.

A bill can experience long delays at this stage; it cannot proceed to the next stage on the same day unless the House so decides, which is rare.

Stage 6. Committee of the whole House

At this stage, the whole House sits as a committee to go through the bill clause by clause and introduce amendments. This stage is a continuation of the second reading, with the same sources of information.

Stage 7. Third reading

This stage usually immediately follows stage 6, at the same sitting or on a day requested by the sponsor. Amendments may be introduced. Unless issues are raised, this stage proceeds quickly, and the bill is finally passed by the House. The speaker forwards the bill to the president for assent within 7 days of the third reading.

Stage 8. Presidential assent

The president is required to assent to the bill within 14 days of receiving it from the speaker. If he or she has reservations, it may be referred back for reconsideration. Stakeholders may ask the President not to assent to a bill if it contains provisions that will negatively affect society. Information about this stage can be obtained from:

- the Speaker's Office;
- the Cabinet's Office;
- the *Kenya Gazette*.

Source: K. Wachira, personal communication, 2012.

4.4 Design and convey effective messages

Once the key decision-makers and other targets of the advocacy campaign have been identified, a communication strategy can be devised to deliver the campaign message effectively. The message and the strategy depend on the recipient. Communication can be:

- face-to-face;
- by policy briefs and technical proposals;
- in workshops and meetings;
- through the social media, such as blogs, social networks and e-mail;
- through the media, including newspapers, television and radio;
- through private media, such as newsletters and web sites;
- on billboards and advertisements.

Box 4.2 illustrates how media can be a forum for victims of road traffic crashes to advocate for legislative change. Box 4.3 illustrates how one nongovernmental organization in Mexico has advocated successfully for legislative changes using various communication strategies, including interviews, workshops and the media.

4.5 Cultivate policy champions, and build strong partnerships

Bringing about legislative change usually requires a 'policy champion' and building partnerships. A contact in parliament or with access to parliamentarians can be useful; for example, a parliamentarian can sponsor a private member's bill, and ministry personnel can request or support a bill. Cultivating a 'policy champion' involves identifying a person who is willing and able to sponsor the desired change and to act as the main resource on the issue. Developing such a relationship takes time and a reputation based on expertise, previous successes and other factors.

It is equally important to build partnerships. No individual or organization has all the resources necessary to advocate for legislative or regulatory change, and partnerships can be formed to complement individuals' strengths and weaknesses. Partnerships should be strategic and time-limited if necessary, and each partner should have a specific and clearly defined role in influencing legislative or regulatory change.

4.6 Create an action plan, implement and monitor progress

A well formulated action plan will help guide an advocacy campaign to a successful conclusion. It should serve as a tool for monitoring progress; it should not be fixed but should be reviewed periodically to determine whether it should be revised or replaced. Frequent consultation with partners on its content will ensure that the activities are relevant and problems are anticipated, as more stakeholders become involved and new information and resources become available.

In March 2010, the United Nations General Assembly adopted resolution 64/255 (3) proclaiming the period 2011–2020 as the Decade of Action for Road Safety, with the goal of stabilizing and reducing the forecasted prevalence of road-traffic fatalities around the world. While some countries already have a plan to reduce fatalities, others are using the Decade of Action to formulate and to implement a plan. The process may include the following:

- clearly define the issue;
- collect and analyse data;
- set advocacy goals and objectives;
- identify the targets of the message;
- prepare the messages, including counter-messages, and select the channels of communication;
- identify resources;
- form a network to build, solidify and maintain partnerships as needed;
- implement the advocacy plan;
- monitor the results.

Box 4.2 Using print media to advocate for legislative change: a victim's perspective

THE FOLLOWING IS AN ARTICLE written by a graduate of Wellesley College, USA, who was a volunteer for an international development organization, BRAC International in Uganda and who was injured in a crash, in which she personalizes road traffic crashes and advocates for legislative changes in Uganda.

'I was going to start with a description of October 8, 2010 but I have no recollection of that fateful day, even though I have heard many accounts of it. I was on the pillion of a motorcycle taxi in Uganda, where they have two-wheeler taxis called boda-bodas.

I was with a friend who is tragically no longer alive. I chose to sit in the middle and that ended up saving my life. We had found a safe boda driver and my friend and I were headed to a nightclub on a Friday night, when a speeding car hit us from behind. Neither of us was wearing a helmet since it was inconvenient to carry a helmet around when all you wanted to do was dance the night away in Uganda's nightclubs. My friend wasn't wearing a helmet, even though he owned one. I chose not to buy a helmet though I had seen a motorcycle taxi accident the very week of my own accident. I thought those kind of horrific incidents only happened to others. It could never happen to me. I am lucky that I lived to find out that it could.

If only Uganda had passed a law making it mandatory for everybody to wear helmets while riding two-wheelers. Now, we must make sure that the Delhi government does not make the same error, and demand that Delhi too enforce such a law. Helmets were originally mandatory for all in Delhi. Apparently, some Sikh groups raised an objection that Sikh women should not be forced to wear helmets; since it is impossible to differentiate between Sikh and non-Sikh women, the Delhi government has exempted women from wearing helmets. The result is that a majority of women in the city do not wear helmets when riding two-wheelers.

Imagine my reaction when I see women on two-wheelers with their heads exposed. I want to roll down my window and say, "You could be in an accident, and yes, it could actually happen to you." I want to open my car door and try to get out, only to have them see that I can't, not without help. Seeing my limited mobility ought to convince them to wear a helmet.

You would think that given that my accident happened in 2010, I would be completely recovered by now. I wish that were true. My bodily injuries have indeed healed, but the part of my brain that was injured will remain so. The boda driver suffered only bodily injuries that naturally healed; he was saved from a head injury because of his helmet. I had a brain injury because I chose to look pretty that day. I have learnt my lesson. I had a year of looking very pretty indeed with my head completely shaved for head surgery. I do not enjoy telling this tale. I am doing so because I believe I experienced this horror for a reason: to save others' lives.

My choice of not wearing a helmet didn't only affect me; it affected all my loved ones. My parents' lives have completely changed, because now they can rarely go out together. They make sure one of them is always home to look after me. Yet, they do it without complaint. My 22-year-old brother has chosen to work from home so as to stay close to the family and lend a helping hand. He's supposed to be the younger sibling and I am supposed to take care of him, not the other way round!

Before the accident, I used to ask my friends "what if" questions. It's ironic that I asked my boyfriend, "What if I got into an accident and for the operation the doctors shaved my head. Would you still be with me?" I am lucky that I lived to find out he wasn't fibbing when he said, "Yeah, of course."

I do not take these decisions lightly. Most people don't have loved ones who are willing or able to sacrifice so much, not to mention the ability to pay for quality healthcare. I wish that I could turn back time and go back and wear a helmet. My life would have been much better, as well as the lives of those near and dear to me. Even if the person you are with is a responsible driver, wear a helmet for precaution, as others on the road might not be as responsible.

Count yourself lucky that you have an able body and start protecting your head while you still have the chance. That's an order from someone who made the mistake and is now paying a heavy price.'

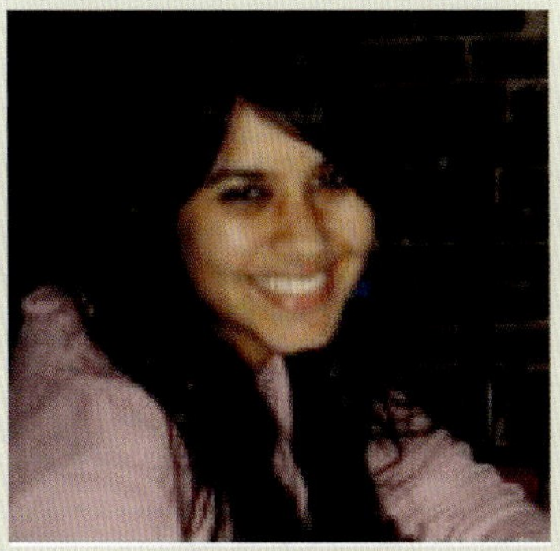

Source: reference *(4)*.

Box 4.3 Advocating for legislative change related to drinking and driving in Mexico

VICTIMAS DE VIOLENCIA VIAL (VIVIAC) operates in the Mexican State of Jalisco. Since its establishment as a nongovernmental organization in 2009, it has used a combination of tactics to influence revision of the Jalisco's legislation on drinking and driving. As it is an association of victims, it provides opportunities for victims and their families to share their personal stories with influential groups in society.

VIVIAC has led a drive to take the road safety cause to state and local legislatures. Under the banner 'Legislando para la Vida' or 'Legislating for Life', VIVIAC describes the nature and consequences of road traffic injuries for individuals to promote stronger road safety legislation, including on drinking and driving. VIVIAC regularly organizes interviews with victims and their families which are disseminated by the broadcast and print media, so that the public hears at first hand from victims about the devastation caused by road traffic crashes and the long-term impacts on their lives. These provide an opportunity to educate the public about the need for stricter laws and law enforcement.

VIVIAC also invites representatives of other nongovernmental organizations, concerned citizens and the media to join 'citizen observatories', in which victims of road traffic crashes and their families join the police in conducting breath tests on drivers. This is one component of a broader campaign to end drinking and driving. In September 2010, with the backing of the three main political parties, the State of Jalisco revised downwards the upper limit of the permitted blood alcohol concentration from 0.15 g/dl to 0.05 g/dl, for the general population, and set a blood alcohol limit of 0.00 g/dl for drivers of public transport vehicles. The new legislation also imposes more severe penalties for those who break the law. Owing in part to advocacy by VIVIAC and the other nongovernmental organizations that comprise the 'Colectivo Ciudadano' (Citizens' Collective), the number of fatalities due to drinking and driving has decreased since the law was enacted. With support from various government ministries, VIVIAC and its partners are organizing advocacy on other issues, such as wearing seat-belts, using child restraints and wearing motorcycle helmets.

Source: reference *(2)*.

These elements need not be completed in the order listed; however, all of them are necessary for a solid advocacy plan. The plan of action should include sufficient detail, milestones and entities but must also be flexible enough to allow for change with circumstances. The plan should include:

- the activities to be conducted;
- the stakeholders who will be involved;
- the responsible agencies, including a lead agency;
- the main 'deliverables';
- timetables and milestones; and
- the resources required.

Ideally, a lead agency will be in charge of the plan and monitor progress in achieving the objectives. If the legislative change involves input from several agencies, each might prepare its own action plan, with an agreed format and timetable for reporting to the lead agency to ensure that the overall plan remains up to date.

4.7 References

1. Richardson Y. Leadership for policy advocacy: keys to achieving success. Paper presented at the WHO Workshop on Road Safety for Lawyers, Geneva, Switzerland, 7-9 August 2012 (unpublished paper).

2. *Advocating for road safety and road traffic victims: a guide for nongovernmental organizations.* Geneva, World Health Organization, 2012.

3. Resolution A/RES/64/255. Improving Global Road Safety. Sixty-fourth session of the United Nations General Assembly, New York, 10 May 2010 (http://www.un.org/en/ga/64/resolutions.shtml, accessed 6 June 2013).

4. Mohan T. Because accidents don't happen only to others. *The Indian Express,* 22 June 2012..

CONCLUSION

Road traffic crashes are one of the leading causes of death and will contribute even more to the number of deaths in years to come if nothing is done. Countries that have been successful in reducing the carnage of road traffic crashes have done so by enacting comprehensive legislation backed by consistent enforcement and social marketing campaigns to bring about change. Yet, many countries lack comprehensive national road safety legislation.

Some, mainly high-income, countries have reduced the numbers of road traffic-related injuries and fatalities through effective road safety programmes, which have included legislative change. Technical knowledge is available both globally and nationally to support the drafting and implementing of comprehensive laws, which can be used by countries embarking on road safety legislative reform.

Passing and implementing comprehensive laws is challenging and time-consuming, and the process is hindered by many factors, such as lack of political will, institutional inertia, lack of resources and competing problems at national level. These hurdles can be overcome by strong advocacy and vigilance in seizing opportunities for advocacy to include road safety in public discourse, such as a change in administration.

This manual provides a road map to achieve comprehensive legislation related to the five main risk factors for road traffic injuries—speed, seat-belts, child restraints, drinking and driving, and motorcycle helmets—as well as in the area of post-crash care. It provides:

- the basic steps that countries can use to develop an understanding of the framework within which legislative change happens;
- processes by which to assess and evaluate existing legislation in order to identify gaps and loopholes;
- links to information resources such as international agreements and evidence-based guidance which can be used to inform the development of comprehensive national legislation;
- steps to advocate for such change.

Annex of laws

Annex of laws

A.1 Speed

The following text is an excerpt from Kenya's Traffic Act, Chapter 403, which covers speeding laws. It was amended in 2012 by an act of parliament to include additional provisions concerning penalties for noncompliance with speeding regulations.

The Traffic Act, Chapter 403

Section 42. (1) - No person shall drive, or, being the owner or person in charge of a vehicle, cause or permit any other person to drive, a vehicle on a road at a speed greater than such speed as may be prescribed as the maximum speed for that class of vehicle.

(2) - On a vehicle subject to a speed restriction under subsection (1) except a vehicle registered as a motor-car or motor-cycle or a private hire vehicle, there shall be painted or affixed to the rear, as close as possible to the rear number plate and so as to be clearly legible to a person within ten metres of the rear of the vehicle, a mark in the prescribed form indicating its maximum permitted speed in kilometres per hour.

(3) - No person shall drive, or, being the owner or person in charge of a vehicle, cause or permit any other person to drive, any vehicle at a speed exceeding fifty kilometres per hour on any road within the boundaries of any trading centre, township, municipality or city:

Provided that the highway authority shall erect and maintain traffic signs as prescribed so as plainly to indicate to drivers entering or leaving such roads or areas where the fifty kilometre per hour speed limit restriction begins and ends.

(4) - Notwithstanding subsections (1) and (3), it shall be lawful for the Minister—

(a) to impose on any road such lower limit of speed as it considers necessary in circumstances when, by reason of repairs, reconstruction or damage to the road or the condition of the road, any lower limit of speed is necessary for the public-safety or to prevent damage to the road:

Provided that such lower limit shall be imposed only for such period as is necessary to carry out repairs or reconstruction or until the condition of the road is satisfactory;

(b) to impose on any road or area, either permanently or for such time as he considers appropriate, such lower limit of speed as may be necessary to prevent damage to the road or for the safety of the public having regard to any permanent or temporary hazards, the alignment or characteristics of the road, the width of streets, nature of traffic or general development of the area:

Provided that, in any case whilst such lower limit is in force under this subsection, indication of the maximum speed permitted shall be given by prescribed traffic signs erected and maintained so as plainly to indicate to drivers entering or leaving such restricted road where the lower speed limit begins and ends.

(4A) The Minister may by notice in the Gazette delegate the power conferred by subsection (4) to a highway authority or other public body.

The Traffic Act, Chapter 403 Section 43—Penalties in relation to speed, as amended by The Traffic (Amendment) (No.2) Act, 2012

11. Section 43 ... (1) Any person who contravenes or fails to comply with any of the provisions of section 42 shall be guilty of an offence and liable to a fine of not exceeding one hundred thousand shillings.

(2) A first or second conviction for an offence under this section shall not render the offender liable to be disqualified for holding or obtaining a licence for a longer period than, in the case of a first conviction, one month, or in the case of a second conviction, three months:

Provided that, if the offender has been convicted of reckless or dangerous driving within the three years immediately preceding the date of his conviction for an offence under this section, such previous conviction shall be treated for the purposes of this subsection as if it had been a conviction for an offence under this section.

(3) A person charged with the offence of driving a motor vehicle of any class or description on a road at a speed greater than the maximum speed allowed shall not be liable to be convicted solely on the evidence of one witness to the effect that in the opinion of the witness the person charged was driving the vehicle at such greater speed.

15. Section 47 ... (1) Any person who drives a motor vehicle on a road recklessly, or at speed, or in a manner which is dangerous to the public, having regard to all the circumstances of the case, including the nature, condition and use of the road and the amount of traffic which is at the time or which might reasonably be expected to be on the road, is guilty of an offence and liable—

(a) for a first conviction, to a fine not exceeding one hundred thousand shillings, or to imprisonment for a term not exceeding two years, and

(b) for a second or subsequent conviction, to a fine not exceeding three hundred thousand shillings, or imprisonment for a term not exceeding one year, and the court shall exercise the power conferred by Part VIII of cancelling any driving licence or provisional driving licence held by the offender and declaring the offender disqualified for holding or obtaining a driving licence for a period of two years starting from the date of conviction or the end of any prison sentence imposed under this section, whichever is later.

Section 49. The principal Act is amended by inserting the following new schedule—

Schedule (s.117A)

Description of offence		*Demerit points*
Exceeding the prescribed speed limit		
(i)	By 10 to 20 Kph	2
(ii)	By 21 to 30 Kph	4
(iii)	By 31 Kph or more	6

References *(1, 2)*.

A.2 Drink–driving

India's Motor Vehicles Act of 1988 includes provisions on drinking and driving, which among other things specify blood alcohol limits and how the drink-driving laws are to be enforced. The relevant sections are reproduced below.

The Motor Vehicles Act of 1988

185. Driving by a drunken person or by a person under the influence of drugs.—Whoever, while driving, or attempting to drive, a motor vehicle,—

1[(a) has, in his blood, alcohol exceeding 30 mg. per 100 ml. of blood detected in a test by a breath analyser, or]

(b) is under this influence of a drug to such an extent as to be incapable of exercising proper control over the vehicle, shall be punishable for the first offence with imprisonment for a term which may extend to six months, or with fine which may extend to two thousand rupees, or with both; and for a second or subsequent offence, if committed within three years of the commission of the previous similar offence, with imprisonment for a term which may extend to two years, or with fine which may extend to three thousand rupees, or with both.

Explanation — For the purposes of this section, the drug or drugs specified by the Central Government in this behalf, by notification in the Official Gazette, shall be deemed to render a person incapable of exercising proper control over a motor vehicle.

203. Breath tests.—1[(1) A police officer in uniform or an officer of the Motor Vehicles Department, as may be authorised in this behalf by that Department, may require any person driving or attempting to drive a motor vehicle in a public place to provide one or more specimens of breath for breath test there or nearby, if such police officer or officer has any reasonable cause to suspect him of having committed an offence under section 185:

Provided that requirement for breath test shall be made (unless, it is made) as soon as reasonably practicable after the commission of such offence.]

(2) - If a motor vehicle is involved in an accident in a public place and a police officer in uniform has any reasonable cause to suspect that the person who was driving the motor vehicle at the time of the accident had alcohol in his blood or that he was driving under the influence of a drug referred to in section 185 he may require the person so driving the motor vehicle, to provide a specimen of his breath for a breath test:

(a) in the case of a person who is at a hospital as an indoor patient, at the hospital;

(b) in the case of any other person, either at or near the place where the requirement is made, or, if the police officer thinks fit, at a police station specified by the police officer:

Provided that a person shall not be required to provide such a specimen while at a hospital as an indoor patient if the registered medical practitioner in immediate charge of his case is not first notified of the proposal to make the requirement or objects to the provision of a specimen on the ground that its provision or the requirement to provide it would be prejudicial to the proper care or treatment of the patient.

(3) - If it appears to a police officer in uniform, in consequence of a breath test carried out by him on any person under sub-section (1) or sub-section (2) that the device by means of which the test has been carried out indicates the presence of alcohol in the person's blood, the police officer may arrest that person without warrant except while that person is at a hospital as an indoor patient.

(4) - If a person, required by a police officer under sub-section (1) or sub-section (2) to provide a specimen of breath for a breath test, refuses or fails to do so and the police officer has reasonable cause to suspect him of having alcohol in his blood, the police officer may arrest him without warrant except while he is at a hospital as an indoor patient.

(5) - A person arrested under this section shall while at a police station, be given an opportunity to provide a specimen of breath for a breath test there.

(6)- The results of a breath test made in pursuance of the provisions of this section shall be admissible in evidence.

Explanation— For the purposes of this section "breath test", means a test for the purpose of obtaining an indication of the presence of alcohol in a person's blood carried out on one or more specimens of breath provided by that person, by means of a device of a type approved by the Central Government by notification in the Official Gazette, for the purpose of such a test.

204. Laboratory test.—(1) - A person who has been arrested under section 203 may, while at a police station be required by a police officer to provide to such registered medical practitioner as may be produced by such police officer, a specimen of his blood for a laboratory test if,

(a) it appears to the police officer that the device, by means of which breath test was taken in relation to such person, indicates the presence of alcohol in the blood of such person, or

(b) such person, when given the opportunity to submit to a breath test, has refused, omitted or failed to do so:

Provided that where the person required to provide such specimen is a female and the registered medical practitioner produced by such police officer is a male medical practitioner, the specimen shall be taken only in the presence of a female, whether a medical practitioner or not.

(2) - A person while at a hospital as an indoor patient may be required by a police officer to provide at the hospital a specimen of his blood for a laboratory test:

(a) if it appears to the police officer that the device by means of which test is carried out in relation to the breath of such person indicates the presence of alcohol in the blood of such person, or

(b) if the person having been required, whether at the hospital or elsewhere, to provide a specimen of breath for a breath test, has refused, omitted or failed to do so and a police officer has reasonable cause to suspect him of having alcohol in his blood:

Explanation—For the purposes of this section, "laboratory test" means the analysis of a specimen of blood made at a laboratory established, maintained or recognised by the Central Government or a State Government.

Provided that a person shall not be required to provide a specimen of his blood for a laboratory test under this sub-section if the registered medical practitioner in immediate charge of his case is not first notified of the proposal to make the requirement or objects to the provision of such specimen on the ground that its provision or the requirement to provide it would be prejudicial to the proper care or treatment of the patient.

(3) - The results of a laboratory test made in pursuance of this section shall be admissible in evidence.

205. Presumption of unfitness to drive.—In any proceeding for an offence punishable under section 185 if it is proved that the accused when requested by a police officer at any time so to do, had refused, omitted or failed to consent to the taking of or providing a specimen of his breath for a breath test or a specimen of his blood for a laboratory test, his refusal, omission or failure may, unless reasonable cause therefor is shown, be presumed to be a circumstance supporting any evidence given on behalf of the prosecution, or rebutting any evidence given on behalf of the defence, with respect to his condition at that time.

Reference *(3)*.

A.3 Motorcycle helmets

An excerpt of the motorcycle helmet law and administrative regulations on penalties in Viet Nam is shown below. The law defines the term motorcycle—including electric motorcycles— and limits the number and age of passengers who can be transported on a motorcycle. Viet Nam has continually reviewed and improved its motorcycle helmet law since it was first enacted in 1995: helmet-wearing has been made compulsory for all riders and passengers on all roads; penalties for noncompliance have increased substantially; helmet standards for adults and children have been set and revised. The law has been further strengthened by requiring compulsory helmet strapping, and the government is examining how to ensure that helmets worn meet the national quality standards.

Law on Land Traffic 2008

Article 30. Operators of, people sitting on motorbikes, mopeds

1. Operators of motorized two-wheelers or mopeds may each only carry one adult and one child at most; in case of carrying sick persons for emergency or escorting criminals, they may each carry two adults in cases:

a) To carry the sick person to emergency unit;

b) To escort the person violating legislation;

c) Children under 14 years of age.

2. The persons operating or sitting on motorized two-wheelers, motorized three-wheelers or mopeds must wear safety helmets buckled properly.

Decree on Regulations on Penalty Settlement of Administrative Violation in the Field of Road Traffic

Chapter I. General Provisions

...

Article 3. Word interpretation

3. Types of motorbike-like vehicles are road vehicles driven by engines, with two or three wheels and their cylinder capacities of more than 50 cm^3, and with the highest design speed of higher than 50 km per hour and its maximum total weight of 400 kg.

4. Electric motorbike is a vehicle with two wheels moving by an electric engine, with its highest design speed of higher than 50 km per hour.

5. Moped (including electric bicycle) is a type of two wheel non-motorized vehicles with engine mounted, the highest design speed of less than 30 km per hour and which can be moved forward by pedalling when the engine is turned off.

6. Types of moped-like vehicles, excluding those stated in Item 5 of this Article are road transport vehicles operating by engines with two or three wheels with the highest design speed of or less than 50 km per hour.

Chapter II. Acts of Administrative Violation, Forms and Rates for Fine

Section 1. Violations of Road Traffic Rules

Article 9. Penalty Settlement on driver(s), person(s) sitting on the motorbike(s), mopeds (including electric motorcycles), and other types of motorbike-like vehicles, moped-like vehicles who violate road traffic rules

...

3. Pecuniary fine from 100,000VND to 200,000VND for any of the violation acts below:

i) The driver, person sitting on the vehicle do not wear helmet(s) or wear helmet(s) without fastening its chin-strap properly while participating in traffic;

...

k) Carry a person sitting on the vehicle without wearing helmet or wearing helmet without fastening its chin-strap properly, except the circumstances of carrying the person to emergency treatment, carrying an under-6 child or escorting the person with law violation act; ...

References *(4, 5)*.

A.4 Seat-belts

The excerpt below is taken from the sections of Jamaica's Road Traffic Act that deal with the fitting and wearing of seat-belts.

Road Traffic Act, Sections 43A and 43B

Vehicles to be equipped with seat-belts. 13/1999 s.2

43A. (1) Subject to subsections (2) - and (3), - a motor vehicle shall not be used on a road unless it is equipped with seat-belts:

(a) in the case of trucks which are constructed to carry passengers as specified in paragraph (b) of section 11(1), on the front seat only;

(b) in the case of motor cars, private motor cars and invalid carriages as specified in paragraphs (c), (d) and (f), respectively of section 11(1), on the front seat and rear seat;

(c) in the case of public passenger vehicles as specified in section 60(1), that is to say:

(i) stage carriages as specified in paragraph a), on the front seat only;

(ii) express carriages as specified in paragraph (b), on the front seat only;

(iii) contract carriages (except trucks) as specified in paragraph (c), on the front seat and rear seat;

(iv) hackney carriages as specified in paragraph (d), on the front seat and rear seat.

(2) - The seat-belts mentioned in subsection (1) shall be of such shape, quality, construction, installation or assembly as may be prescribed.

(3) - Where a motor vehicle specified in paragraph (c), (d) or (f) of section 11(1) is constructed with a front seat, a rear seat and any other seat, all the seats shall be equipped with seat-belts.

(4) A person who uses a motor vehicle on any road in contravention of subsection (1) or (3) commits an offence and is liable on summary conviction before a Resident Magistrate:

(a) in the case of a first offence, to a fine not exceeding two thousand dollars;

(b) in the case of a second or subsequent offence, to a fine not exceeding five thousand dollars.

Drivers, etc. of motor vehicles to wear seat-belts . 13/1999 s.2.

43B. (1) - Subject to subsection (2), every person who, on any road:

(a) drives a motor vehicle specified in paragraph (b), (c), (d) or (f) of section 11(1);

(b) rides in a motor vehicle specified in paragraph (c), (d) or (f) of section 11(1);

(c) rides in the front seat of-

(i) a truck as specified in paragraph (b) of section 11(1);

(ii) a stage carriage as specified in paragraph a) of section 60(1);

(iii) an express carriage as specified in paragraph (b) of section 60(1), shall wear a seat-belt.

(2) Subsection (1) shall not apply to:

(a) a child who wears or is conveyed in a child restraint system;

(b) a driver of a motor vehicle while performing a manoeuvre which includes reversing;

(c) any person who holds a valid certificate of exemption prescribed by the Minister and signed by a registered medical practitioner as defined under section 2 of the Medical Act;

(d) a person riding in a vehicle while it is being used for fire brigade or police purposes;

(e) a person driving or riding in a vehicle constructed or adapted for the delivery of goods or mail to consumers or premises, as the case may be, while engaged in the delivery to, or collection of such goods or mail from, consumers or premises, not further than sixty metres from each other.

...

(3) A person who drives or rides in a motor vehicle in contravention of the provisions of this section commits an offence and is liable on summary conviction before a Resident Magistrate:

(a) in the case of a first offence, to a fine not exceeding two thousand dollars;

(b) in the case of a second or subsequent offence, to a fine not exceeding five thousand dollars.

Reference *(6)*.

A.5 Post-crash care

Excerpts from various laws from Australia, Canada, India, South African and the USA, as well as European recommendations on measures relating to the provision of first aid, are presented below.

A.5.a Duty to provide assistance in road traffic crashes

The Road Transport (Safety and Traffic Management) Act 1999 in New South Wales, Australia, includes a requirement that the driver of a vehicle involved in a crash that causes death or injury must stop and give all possible assistance. The law covers only people directly involved in the crash.

Duty to stop and give assistance where person killed or injured in road accident

The driver or rider of a vehicle or horse concerned in an accident that occurs because of the presence of the vehicle or horse on a road or road related area and that causes the death of or injury to any person must not knowingly fail to stop and give any assistance that may be necessary and that it is in his or her power to give.

Maximum penalty: 30 penalty units or imprisonment for 18 months or both (in the case of a first offence) or 50 penalty units or imprisonment for 2 years or both (in the case of a second or subsequent offence).

Reference *(7)*.

A.5.b 'Good Samaritan' laws

Some countries have 'good Samaritan' laws that provide protection from liability for people who give assistance to the injured, irrespective of whether the country has a law making it a duty for bystanders to provide assistance in case of an emergency. A 'good Samaritan can be defined generally as as a person (including a medical practitioner) who in good faith and without expectation of payment or reward comes to the aid of an injured person, or person at risk of injury, with assistance or advice' (8). People who fall outside the definition of the law as 'good Samaritan' are generally excluded from protection. Examples of laws which protect bystanders who assist those injured in road traffic crashes from prosecution for damages are provided by the New South Wales Emergency Medical Aid Act (Australia) and British Columbia's Good Samaritan Act (Canada).

Emergency Medical Aid Act 1988

Definition

1. In this Act, 'nurse' means a registered nurse, a nurse practitioner or a temporary certificate holder under the Nursing Profession Act. S .N.W.T.2002,c.11,s.33; S.N.W.T. 2003,c.15,s.75(2).

Protection of certain persons from action

2. Where, in respect of a person who is ill, injured or unconscious as the result of an accident or other emergency,

(a) a medical practitioner or nurse voluntarily renders emergency medical services or first aid assistance, and the services or assistance are not rendered at a hospital or other place having adequate medical facilities and equipment, or

(b) a person other than a medical practitioner or a nurse voluntarily renders emergency first aid assistance, the medical practitioner, nurse or other person is not liable for damages for injuries to or the death of that person alleged to have been caused by an act or omission on the part of the medical practitioner, nurse or other person in rendering the medical services or first aid assistance, unless it is established that the injuries or death were caused by gross negligence on the part of the medical practitioner, nurse or other person. S.N.W.T. 2003,c.15,s.75(3).

Reference *(9)*.

Good Samaritan Act, 1996

No liability for emergency aid unless gross negligence

1. A person who renders emergency medical services or aid to an ill, injured or unconscious person, at the immediate scene of an accident or emergency that has caused the illness, injury or unconsciousness, is not liable for damages for injury to or death of that person caused by the person's act or omission in rendering the medical services or aid unless that person is grossly negligent.

Exceptions

2. Section 1 does not apply if the person rendering the medical services or aid;

Annex of laws

(a) is employed expressly for that purpose, or

(b) does so with a view to gain.

Health Care (Consent) and Care Facility (Admission) Act

3. The Health Care (Consent) and Care Facility (Admission) Act does not affect anything in this Act.

References *(9,10)*.

A.5.c Ambulance services

The Ontario Ambulance Act places the responsibility on the Minister of Health to establish, administer and regulate ambulance services in Ontario, Canada, including cooperating with other entities to meet the requirements of the Act The relevant sections of the Act are reproduced below.

Part II. Provincial responsibilities

Ontario Ambulance Act, R.S.O. 1999

...

Administration of Act

2. The Minister is responsible for the administration and enforcement of this Act. R.S.O. 1990, c. A.19, s. 2.

Advisory council

3. The Minister may establish an advisory council for the purpose of advising the Minister on matters respecting the provision of ambulance services in the Province. 1999, c. 12, Sched. J, s. 2.

Functions of Minister

4. (1) - The Minister has the duty and the power,

(a) to ensure the existence throughout Ontario of a balanced and integrated system of ambulance services and communication services used in dispatching ambulances;

(b) Repealed: 1997, c. 30, Sched. A, s. 5 (2);

(c) to establish, maintain and operate communication services, alone or in co-operation with others, and to fund such services;

(d) to establish standards for the management, operation and use of ambulance services and to ensure compliance with those standards;

(e) to monitor, inspect and evaluate ambulance services and investigate complaints respecting ambulance services; and

(f) to fund and ensure the provision of air ambulance services. R.S.O. 1990, c. A.19, s. 4 *(1)*; 1997, c. 30, Sched. A, s. 5 *(1-4)*; 1999, c. 12, Sched. J, s. 3.

Powers of Minister

(2) The Minister has, in addition to the powers under subsection (1), the power,

(a) to establish and operate, alone or in co-operation with one or more organizations, institutes and centres for the training of personnel for ambulance services and communication services;

(b) to require hospitals to establish, maintain and operate ambulance services and communication services;

(c) to establish regions and districts for the purposes of ambulance services and communication services; and

(d) to designate hospitals as base hospitals that shall monitor the quality of the care provided by ambulance services in the regions and districts established by the Minister under clause (c) and perform such other functions as may be assigned to them by regulation. 1997, c. 30, Sched. A, s. 5 (5).

Reference *(11)*.

A.5.d First-aid training and kits

The United Nations Economic Commission for Europe has produced a series of recommendations relating to the issue of first aid in the context of road safety. These are included in the 2009 Consolidated Resolution on Road Traffic. The sections that relate to first-aid training for drivers and the composition of first-aid kits are presented below.

Consolidated Resolution on Road Traffic, 14 August 2009

2.1.2 First-aid training

(a) Appropriate measures shall be taken to ensure that candidates for driver's licences receive proper training concerning their conduct at an accident site, so as to minimize the hazard to life or health at the scene;

b) Drivers and other people should be encouraged to acquire first aid training on a voluntary basis through courses or through mass media or any other appropriate means.

5.3.2 First–aid kit

5.3.2.1 General recommendations

A first-aid kit should be placed in all motor vehicles of categories B, C and D and their subcategories, as set out in annex 6 to the Convention on Road Traffic of 1968.

The content of the kit should be adapted according to the category of vehicle considered or the particular use made of the vehicle, such as the transport of dangerous goods.

For vehicles in category B, the first-aid kit should be:

(a) simple, appropriate and safe to use;

(b) affordable;

(c) easily replenished locally, including the inclusion of a limited number of products with expiry dates; and

(d) adapted to local practices and conditions.

5.3.2.2 Recommendations concerning the container of the first-aid kit and its contents

(a) Container

The container should hold the items detailed below and should be designed to protect them against impact, dust and water. It should be of distinctive colour and/or bear a distinctive sign. It should be easy to open and close. It should also contain compartments to hold different items. It may take the form of a shoulder bag, backpack or box.

(b) Contents

The first-aid kit for category B vehicles should contain at least the following articles, in order to enable persons not formally trained in medicine, but having basic first-aid training, to perform the actions required to save or protect lives:

Reference *(12)*.

Action	Content	Description	Quantity
Reminders for actions to assist victims	Information booklet: - Emergency numbers - List of kit contents - Instructions on how to use the kit	Pocket-sized format More graphics than text	1
Protection of victims against cold or heat	Article to limit differences between the victim's body temperature and the outside temperature.	Isothermal rescue blanket: About 210 cm x 160 cm Very bright colour	1
Controlling external bleeding	Article to protect rescuer's hands against contact with victim's blood	Pair of gloves: non-sterile, latex-free, large	1
	Article to absorb blood loss during clotting and to maintain sufficient local pressure to control bleeding	Compress, gauze, non-sterile (10 x 10, absorbent gauze, 100% cotton, woven, 17 threads/cm^2)	5
		Bandage, gauze, non-sterile (10 cm x 4 m, 100% cotton)	1
		Safety pins or adhesive tape (5 cm x 10 m, capable of being torn by hand, high cutaneous tolerance, waterproof, microporous, with strong adherence and non-damaging for the skin when removed)	2 or 1
	Article to stop major bleeding in the event of serious injuries to a limb	Rubber tourniquet	1
Care of skin wounds	Antiseptic protective barrier to prevent or limit possible infectious contamination	Single-use doses of non-iodized antiseptic, e.g. chlorhexidine 0.05%.	4
		Compress, gauze, non-sterile (10 x 10 cm, absorbent gauze, 10% cotton, woven, 17 threads/cm2)	2
		Adhesive dressings	1 small box of assorted sizes, or adhesive dressing bandage (6 cm x 5 m, 1 roll)
Stabilize bone in joint trauma	Material to restrict movement of the wound	Triangular bandage (136 x 96 x 96 cm, 100% cotton or viscose)	2
Artificial respiration	Means to restrict direct contact between rescuer and victim during mouth-to-mouth resuscitation	Face shield or pocket mask	1
Miscellaneous	Sharp instrument to cut things (seat belt, clothes, bandages, dressings)	Pair of curved scissors (unhardened, non-magnetic steel)	1
	Means of illuminating the scene and the victim	Pocket torch	1
	Notebook	Pocket-sized	1
	Pen or pencil		1

A.5.e Duty to provide emergency stabilization services

In the USA, federal law requires that facilities have emergency medical departments as a condition for receiving federal funds, to screen and stabilize any person who presents to the emergency department. Similarly, India's Clinical Establishments Registration and Regulation Act of 2010 makes it mandatory for all clinical establishments to provide medical care and treatment to stabilize any person in an emergency condition and authorizes the regulatory authority to impose a fine for noncompliance. Excerpts from both acts are given below.

The Federal Emergency Medical Treatment and Active Labor Act

§ 1395dd. Examination and treatment for emergency medical conditions and women in labor

(a) Medical screening requirement

In the case of a hospital that has a hospital emergency department, if any individual (whether or not eligible for benefits under this subchapter) comes to the emergency department and a request is made on the individual's behalf for examination or treatment for a medical condition, the hospital must provide for an appropriate medical screening examination within the capability of the hospital's emergency department, including ancillary services routinely available to the emergency department, to determine whether or not an emergency medical condition (within the meaning of subsection (e)(1) of this section) exists.

...

(c) Restricting transfers until individual stabilized

...

(1) Rule

If an individual at a hospital has an emergency medical condition which has not been stabilized (within the meaning of subsection (e)(3)(B) of this section), the hospital may not transfer the individual unless—

(A) (i) the individual (or a legally responsible person acting on the individual's behalf) after being informed of the hospital's obligations under this section and of the risk of transfer, in writing requests transfer to another medical facility,

(ii) a physician (within the meaning of section 1395x(r)(1) of this title) has signed a certification that based upon the information available at the time of transfer, the medical benefits reasonably expected from the provision of appropriate medical treatment at another medical facility outweigh the increased risks to the individual and, in the case of labor, to the unborn child from effecting the transfer, or

(iii) if a physician is not physically present in the emergency department at the time an individual is transferred, a qualified medical person (as defined by the Secretary in regulations) has signed a certification described in clause (ii) after a physician (as defined in section 1395x(r)(1) of this title), in consultation with the person, has made the determination described in such clause, and subsequently countersigns the certification; and

(B) the transfer is an appropriate transfer (within the meaning of paragraph (2) to that facility.

A certification described in clause (ii) or (iii) of subparagraph (A) shall include a summary of the risks and benefits upon which the certification is based.

(2) Appropriate transfer

An appropriate transfer to a medical facility is a transfer:

(A) in which the transferring hospital provides the medical treatment within its capacity which minimizes the risks to the individual's health and, in the case of a woman in labor, the health of the unborn child;

(B) in which the receiving facility:

(i) has available space and qualified personnel for the treatment of the individual; and

(ii) has agreed to accept transfer of the individual and to provide appropriate medical treatment;

(C) in which the transferring hospital sends to the receiving facility all medical records (or copies thereof), related to the emergency condition for which the individual has presented, available at the time of the transfer, including records related to the individual's emergency medical condition, observations of signs or symptoms, preliminary diagnosis, treatment provided, results of any tests and the informed written consent or certification (or copy thereof) provided under paragraph (1)(A), and the name and address of any on-call physician (described in subsection (d)(1)(C) of this section) who has refused or failed to appear within a reasonable time to provide necessary stabilizing treatment;

(D) in which the transfer is effected through qualified personnel and transportation equipment, as required including the use of necessary and medically appropriate life support measures during the transfer; and

(E) which meets such other requirements as the Secretary may find necessary in the interest of the health and safety of individuals transferred.

(d) Enforcement

(1) Civil money penalties

(A) A participating hospital that negligently violates a requirement of this section is subject to a civil money penalty of not more than $50,000 (or not more than $25,000 in the case of a hospital with less than 100 beds) for each 8such violation...

(B) Subject to subparagraph (C), any physician who is responsible for the examination, treatment, or transfer of an individual in a participating hospital, including a physician on-call for the care of such an individual, and who negligently violates a requirement of this section, including a physician who:

(i) signs a certification under subsection (c)(1)(A) of this section that the medical benefits reasonably to be expected from a transfer to another facility outweigh the risks associated with the transfer, if the physician knew or should have known that the benefits did not outweigh the risks, or

(ii) misrepresents an individual's condition or other information, including a hospital's obligations under this section, is subject to a civil money penalty of not more than $50,000 for each such violation and, if the violation is gross and flagrant or is repeated, to exclusion from participation in this subchapter and State health care programs...

(C) If, after an initial examination, a physician determines that the individual requires the services of a physician listed by the hospital on its list of on-call physicians (required to be maintained under section 1395cc(a)(1)(I) of this title) and notifies the on-call physician and the on-call physician fails or refuses to appear within a reasonable period of time, and the physician orders the transfer of the individual because the physician determines that without the services of the on-call physician the benefits of transfer outweigh the risks of transfer, the physician authorizing the transfer shall not be subject to a penalty under subparagraph (B). However, the previous sentence shall not apply to the hospital or to the on-call physician who failed or refused to appear.

(2) Civil enforcement

(A) Personal harm

Any individual who suffers personal harm as a direct result of a participating hospital's violation of a requirement of this section may, in a civil action against the participating hospital, obtain those damages available for personal injury under the law of the State in which the hospital is located, and such equitable relief as is appropriate;

(B) Financial loss to other medical facility

Any medical facility that suffers a financial loss as a direct result of a participating hospital's violation of a requirement of this section may, in a civil action against the participating hospital, obtain those damages available for financial loss, under the law of the State in which the hospital is located, and such equitable relief as is appropriate."

Reference (13).

Clinical Establishments Registration and Regulation Act, 2010

The Act provides a legislative framework for the registration and regulation of clinical establishments, including hospitals, maternity homes, nursing homes, dispensaries, clinics and similar facilities with beds that offer diagnosis, treatment or care for illness or injury or pregnancy and laboratories under any recognized system in India. It permits categorization and classification of clinical establishments by their location and the services offered a first step in the creation of a national registry of clinical establishments. The objective of the act is to improve the quality of health services through the National Council for Standards by prescribing minimum standards for facilities and the services they may provide. It also empowers state governments or the registering authority to direct any clinical establishment to furnish details, statistics or any other information.

Chapter II. The National Council for Clinical Establishments

12. Condition for registration. (1) - For registration and continuation, every clinical establishment shall fulfil the following conditions, namely:

...

(ii) the minimum requirement of personnel as may be prescribed;

(iii) provisions for maintenance of records and reporting as may be prescribed;

(iv) such other conditions as may be prescribed.

(2) The clinical establishment shall undertake to provide within the staff and facilities available, such medical examination and treatment as may be required to stabilise the emergency medical condition of any individual who comes or is brought to such clinical establishment.

Reference *(14)*.

A.5.f Victims' Compensation

In South Africa, a portion of the fuel levy goes into a fund that is used to pay compensation in accordance with the Road Accident Fund Act for loss or damage wrongfully caused by the driving of motor vehicles. An excerpt from the Acts is presented below.

Road Accident Fund Act, amended 2005

Establishment of Fund

2. (1) There is hereby established a juristic person to be known as the Road Accident Fund.

(a) Subject to section 28(1), the Multilateral Motor Vehicle Accidents Fund established by the Agreement concluded between the Contracting Parties on 14 February 1989, shall cease to exist, and all money credited to that fund immediately before the commencement of this Act shall vest in the Fund, all assets, liabilities, fights and obligations, existing as well as accruing, of the first-mentioned fund shall devolve upon the Fund, and any reference in any law or document to the said Multilateral Motor Vehicle Accidents Fund shall, unless clearly inappropriate, be construed as a reference to the Fund.

(b) No moneys, duties or fees of office shall be payable by the Fund in respect of any noting or endorsement or any other written alteration which may be necessary in any contract, licence, register or other document by virtue of paragraph (a).

Object of Fund

3. The object of the Fund shall be the payment of compensation in accordance with this Act for loss or damage wrongfully caused by the driving of motor vehicles.

Powers and functions of Fund

4. (1) The powers and functions of the Fund shall include:

(a) the stipulation of the terms and conditions upon which claims for the compensation contemplated in section 3, shall be administered;

(b) the investigation and settling, subject to this Act, of claims arising from loss or damage caused by the driving of a motor vehicle whether or not the identity of the owner or the driver thereof, or the identity of both the owner and the driver thereof, has been established;

(c) the management and utilisation of the money of the Fund for purposes connected with or resulting from the exercise of its powers or the performance of its duties; and

(d) procuring reinsurance for any risk undertaken by the Fund under this Act.

(2) In order to achieve its object, the Fund may:

(a) purchase or otherwise acquire goods, equipment, land, buildings, shares, debentures, stock, securities and all other kinds of movable and immovable property;

(b) sell, lease, mortgage, encumber, dispose of, exchange, cultivate, develop, build upon, improve or in any other way deal with its property;

(c) invest any money not immediately required for the conduct of its business and realise, alter or reinvest such investments or otherwise deal with such money or investments;

(d) borrow money and secure the payment thereof in such manner as it may deem fit;

(e) make donations for research in connection with any matter relating to injuries sustained in motor vehicle accidents on such conditions as it may deem advisable;

(f) draw, draft, accept, endorse, discount, sign and issue promissory notes, bills and other negotiable or transferable instruments, excluding share certificates;

(g) take any other action or steps which are incidental or conducive to the exercise of its powers or the performance of its functions.

(3) In the exercising of the powers conferred on it by this Act, the Fund may deal with any person, partnership, association, company, corporation or other juristic person wherever seated.

Financing of Fund

5. (1) The Fund shall procure the funds it requires to perform its functions:

(a) by way of a fuel levy in respect of all fuel sold within the Republic; and

(b) by raising loans.

(2) There shall be paid into the Fund monthly the amount of money by virtue of the provisions of section 1(2) (a)(ii) of the Central Energy Fund Act, 1977 (Act No. 38 of 1977), calculated for the latest month for which such amount can be calculated, and such payments shall be accompanied by statements reflecting the sale of fuel within the Republic.

Reference *(15)*.

References

1. Government of Kenya. The Traffic Act, Chapter 403, revised edition 2010. Nairobi, National Council for Law Reporting, 2009 (http://www.kenyalaw.org/kenyalaw/klr_home/, accessed 14 January 2013).

2. Government of Kenya. The Traffic (Amendment) (No. 2) Act, November 2012. Nairobi, National Council for Law Reporting, 2012 (http://www.kenyalaw.org/klr/index.php?id=937, accessed 14 January 2013).

3. Supreme Court. Indian Motor Vehicles Act 1988, Section 204. New Delhi (http://indiacode.nic.in/, accessed 9 January 2013).

4. Government of Viet Nam. Law on Land Traffic. Hanoi, 2008.

5. Government of Viet Nam. Decree on regulations on penalty settlement of administrative violation in the field of road traffic. Hanoi, 2010.

6. Government of Jamaica. Road Traffic Act. Section 43A and 43 B, seat-belts and protective helmets (http://moj.gov.jm/laws?title=&field_tags_tid=All&page=16&order=title&sort=asc, accessed 10 January 2013).

7. Government of New South Wales. Road Transport (Safety and Traffic Management) Act 1999, No. 20 Part 5, Division 3, Section 70 (http://www.legislation.nsw.gov.au/maintop/view/inforce/act+20+1999+pt.5-div.3-sec.70+0+N?, accessed 10 January 2013).

8. Bird S. Good Samaritans. Australian Family Physician, 2008; 37:570–571.

9. Government of New South Wales. Emergency Medical Aid Act, R.S.N.W.T. 1988,c.E-4 (http://www.justice.gov.nt.ca/PDF/ACTS/Emerg_Med_Aid.pdf , accessed 10 January 2013).

10. Government of British Columbia. Good Samaritan Act, Chapter 172 (RSBC 1996), Vancouver.

11. Government of Ontario. Ontario Ambulance Act, R.S.O. 1990, Chapter A.19, last amendment: 2009, c. 33, Sched. 18, ss. 1, 17 (2) (http://www.e-laws.gov.on.ca/html/statutes/english/elaws_statutes_90a19_e.htm, accessed 10 January 2013).

12. United Nations Economic Commission for Europe. Consolidated resolution on road traffic, 14 August 2009 (ECE/TRANS/WP.1/123) (http://www.unece.org/trans/roadsafe/wp1fdoc.html, accessed 9 January 2013).

13. United States Government. Title 42 USC, The Public Health and Welfare, Section 1395dd, Washington DC, Government Printing Office (http://www.gpo.gov/fdsys/pkg/USCODE-2011-title42/pdf/USCODE-2011-title42-chap7-subchapXVIII-partE-sec1395dd.pdf, accessed 10 January 2013).

14. Government of India. Clinical Establishments (Registration & Regulation Act), 2010 (http://indiacode.nic.in/, accessed 10 January 2013).

15. Government of South Africa. Road Accident Fund Amendment Act of 2005 (http://www.info.gov.za/gazette/acts/1996/a56-96.htm, accessed 10 January 2013).